Keto Diet Fast

Intermittent Fasting & The Ketogenic Diet; The Secret to Achieving Your Dream Body!

Fitness & Health Fuel

The contents of this book may not be reproduced, duplicated or transmitted without direct written permission from the author.

Under no circumstances will any legal responsibility or blame be held against the publisher for any reparation, damages, or monetary loss due to the information herein, either directly or indirectly.

Legal Notice:

This book is copyright protected. This is only for personal use. You cannot amend, distribute, sell, use, quote or paraphrase any part or the content within this book without the consent of the author.

Disclaimer Notice:

Please note the information contained within this document is for educational and entertainment purposes only. Every attempt has been made to provide accurate, up to date and reliable complete information. No warranties of any kind are expressed or implied. Readers acknowledge that the author is not engaging in the rendering of legal, financial, medical or professional advice. The content of this book has been derived from various sources. Please consult a licensed professional before attempting any techniques outlined in this book.

By reading this document, the reader agrees that under no circumstances are is the author responsible for any losses, direct or indirect, which are incurred as a result of the use of information contained within this document, including, but not limited to, —errors, omissions, or inaccuracies.

© Copyright 2018 Dibbly Publishing.

All rights reserved.

WAIT! Sign Up Now And Get A FREE Bonus!

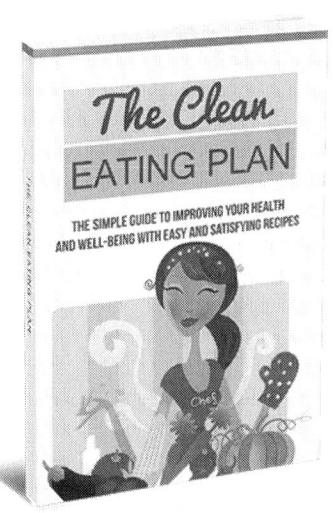

Discover How To Finally Take Control Of Your Diet And Eat Cleaner

- Discover how to eat healthier and cleaner without extra effort

- How your body works and how you can lose weight

- **How to train yourself so that you can eat cleaner forever**

- How to set and achieve your short and long term health goals

- **How to minimize time spent preparing meals**

- And so much more...

https://dibblypublishing.com/fht-bonuses

Contents

INTRODUCTION 1
CHAPTER ONE ABOUT INTERMITTENT FASTING 3
CHAPTER TWO METHODS OF INTERMITTENT FASTING .. 7
    16/8 METHOD 7
    THE 5:2 DIET 8
    FAST-STOP-EAT 9
    ALTERNATE DAY FASTING 10
    SKIPPING MEALS SPONTANEOUSLY 10
CHAPTER THREE BENEFITS OF INTERMITTENT FASTING 13
CHAPTER FOUR WHO SHOULDN'T FAST 17
    PEOPLE WHO CAN FAST 17
    PEOPLE WHO MUST NOT FAST 18
    INTERMITTENT FASTING AND HORMONES 20
CHAPTER FIVE COMMON INTERMITTENT FASTING MISTAKES TO AVOID 25
CHAPTER SIX TRUTH ABOUT BREAKFAST 29
CHAPTER SEVEN POPULAR INTERMITTENT FASTING MYTHS 33
CHAPTER EIGHT ABOUT THE KETOGENIC DIET 39
CHAPTER NINE VARIATIONS OF THE KETO DIET 43
    YOUR VARIATION OF THE KETO DIET 46
    ALTERATIONS NECESSARY FOR CKD 49

Alterations Necessary For TKD 51

CHAPTER TEN BENEFITS OF THE KETOGENIC DIET 55

CHAPTER ELEVEN HOW TO ACHIEVE KETOSIS 61

CHAPTER TWELVE KETO FOOD LIST................................ 63
Eat Freely.. 63
Eat Occasionally 65
Foods To Avoid... 68

CHAPTER THIRTEEN INTERMITTENT FASTING & THE KETOGENIC DIET 71

CHAPTER FOURTEEN TIPS WHILE EATING OUT.............. 75

CHAPTER FIFTEEN CREATE A PLAN 81
Preparation 86

CHAPTER SIXTEEN KETO MEAL PLAN PREP.................... 91
Tips For A Keto Meal Prep 106

CHAPTER SEVENTEEN COMMON KETO MISTAKES TO AVOID 111
Side Effects To Watch Out For And How To Tackle Them 116

CHAPTER EIGHTEEN EXERCISE ON KETO..................... 119

CHAPTER NINETEEN GAIN MUSCLE WHILE FASTING ... 123

CHAPTER TWENTY HOW TO STAY MOTIVATED........... 129
Go 130
Things To Expect.. 134

CHAPTER TWENTY-ONE KETO AND INTERMITTENT FASTING FAQS.. 139

CHAPTER TWENTY-TWO ADDITIONAL TIPS FOR WEIGHT LOSS 153

CHAPTER TWENTY THREE MEAL PLAN 161
Day 1 161
Day 2 161
Day 3 162
Day 4 162
Day 5 163
Day 6 163
Day 7 163

CONCLUSION 165

SOURCES 167

Introduction

I want to thank you for purchasing this book, *'Keto Diet Fast: Intermittent Fasting & The Ketogenic Diet; The Secret to Achieving Your Dream Body!'*

Do you want a diet that will help you shed all those extra pounds and improve your overall health? If yes, then which diet is perfect for you? There are different diets these days, and each claim to be quite helpful. Does it seem overwhelming to select one diet? If yes, then this is the perfect book for you. Intermittent fasting and the ketogenic diet are the two most popular diets these days. These diets are quite effective on their own; however, what will happen if you combine these two diets? Well, that's what this book is all about. In this book, you will learn about the protocols of intermittent fasting, the ketogenic diet and the ways in which you can combine these diets to create a super-diet. The first part of the book covers intermittent fasting, the second portion deals with the ketogenic diet and the third part includes information about a combined diet.

Intermittent fasting is a pattern of eating that oscillates between periods of fasting and eating. If you decide to follow the protocols of intermittent fasting, then you will need to fast for about 16-24 hours. There are different ways to follow intermittent fasting, and you can select a method that suits your needs and requirements. In this book you will learn about intermittent fasting, different methods of intermittent fasting, benefits and some helpful tips to follow this diet.

The ketogenic diet, or the keto diet, is a low-carb and a high-fat diet. The protocols of the keto diet are quite simple. You need to reduce your intake or carbs and, instead, consume naturally fatty foods. On this diet, the primary fuel for the body is fats instead of glucose. Carbs are the main reason for weight gain and, when you cut carbs out of your diet, the process of weight loss accelerates. The keto diet encourages your body to burn fats to generate energy. In this book, you will learn about the keto diet, the benefits it offers, a keto food list, keto myths and different tips to make the keto diet easy.

Apart from this, you will learn about the way in which you can combine the keto diet and intermittent fasting to achieve your weight loss and health goals in 90 days. The steps to create a diet plan, along with the tips to stay motivated, will come in handy when you follow this diet. So, are you ready to turn your life around and want to learn more about these exciting diets? If yes, then let us start without further ado.

Chapter One

About Intermittent Fasting

Intermittent fasting is not a recent craze and is an ancient practice; however, this diet has started to gain popularity in recent times. Intermittent fasting has certainly revolutionized the world of fitness. There are various studies and research that prove that this diet helps with weight loss, improves immunity and boosts the metabolism rate. In this chapter, you will learn what intermittent fasting is all about.

Intermittent fasting might sound slightly technical, but you have probably done this unknowingly. Before you learn what intermittent fasting is about, you must know the difference between fasting and fed states. Whenever you eat after every couple of hours, your body is in a "fed" state. In the fed state, your body will digest, absorb and assimilate nutrients from the food you consume. The main priority of your body in this state is to burn fat. Most of us tend to stay in a fed state throughout the day, except when we sleep. The reason why intermittent fasting provides the benefits it does is that it helps your body enter a fasted state. In a "fasted" state, your body burns fats to provide energy.

Intermittent fasting is a diet that oscillates between

periods of eating and fasting. There are no dietary restrictions that this diet prescribes. Instead, it focuses on the timeframe within when you eat and not what you eat. There are different forms of intermittent fasting. You probably have never given it a conscious thought, but you fast daily. Does that surprise you? Well, take a moment to think about it. You are essentially fasting whenever you sleep. Yes, it might sound silly, but your body fasts while you are asleep. Intermittent fasting is a mere extension of this period of fasting. If you skip your breakfast, have your first meal at noon and the last one at night, your body is on an intermittent fast. In fact, it is one of the most popular methods of intermittent fasting. Essentially, your body is on a fast for about 16 hours in a day and the eating window is restricted to 8 hours. This method of fasting is known as the 16/8 method. In spite of popular notions, intermittent fasting is a simple dieting protocol. Hunger is not difficult to manage and you can tackle it quite easily. It might seem a little tricky, at least initially, however, your body will get used to this diet within no time. You cannot consume anything during the fasting period. The idea of a fast is to not consume any calories for a while, so it means that you can consume anything that is free of calories. Once your body is on a fast, it uses the internal reserves of fat to provide energy.

The concept of fasting is not a new one. In fact, fasting is a concept that humans are quite familiar with. People tend to fast out of necessity or even due to the scarcity of food. People tend to fast for religious reasons as well. For instance, different religions like Hinduism, Buddhism, Islam and Christianity prescribe fasting from time to time. Animals, as well as humans fast during illness as well. There is nothing unnatural or unusual about fasting. Your body, by design, can sustain itself without food for prolonged periods. There are different processes that change in your body whenever you fast. For instance, the levels of blood sugar reduce and the level of insulin decreases. This is desirable if your blood sugar levels are usually high. There is a spurt in the production of human growth hormone as well. There are different beneficial changes that take place in your body whenever you fast; and you will learn about them in the coming chapters.

Chapter Two

Methods of Intermittent Fasting

Intermittent fasting is a popular method of fasting and has various benefits. One of the reasons for the popularity of this diet is its versatility. Intermittent fasting can be practiced in different ways and you can select one that works well for you and suits your needs.

16/8 Method

In this method of intermittent fasting, you need to fast for 16 hours daily. The eating window is therefore restricted to about eight hours. You can squeeze in two or three regular meals during this timeframe. It is quite a simple method to follow. You can perhaps skip breakfast and not munch on any snacks post-dinner. For instance, you can ensure that your last meal is at eight at night and you don't eat anything until noon the following day. It provides your body with the 16-hour fasting window that this diet prescribes. The ideal duration of fast for women is about 14-15 hours. If you are a morning person and are in the habit of having breakfast daily, then it might be slightly difficult initially; however, if you don't mind skipping breakfast, then this is a very simple diet to follow. You can adjust your diet to suit your needs. If you like to exercise in the morning and have a light breakfast, then you can adjust your eating window such that you can have breakfast at 10am and extend the eating window up to 6 in the evening. You can consume water, coffee, green tea and other calorie-free beverages during the fast. It is important that you stay away from all sorts of junk food and eat healthy meals once you break the fast. The 16/8 method will not be of much help if you binge on high-caloric junk foods when you break the fast. Also, it is easier to stick to this diet if you consume foods that are low on carbs and rich in natural fats.

The 5:2 Diet

When you follow this method of intermittent fasting, you need to ensure that your calorie intake on two days of the week is about 500-600 calories and you can eat like you normally do on the other five days in the week. The 5:2 diet is also known as the Fast Diet. The recommended calorie intake for women on the fasting days is 600 calories and that for men is 500 calories. On the days of fast, you can squeeze in two or three small meals of about 200 calories each. This diet is ideal for all those who are averse to the idea of a daily fast. For instance, you can fast on Tuesday and Thursday and eat like you usually do on the other days of the week. It makes sense to not fast on two consecutive days.

Fast-Stop-Eat

In this form of intermittent fasting, you need to fast for 24 hours once or twice a week. You will need to fast for an entire day or 24-hours. For instance, you can start your fast after dinner on one day and fast until dinner on the following day so, you will essentially fast for 24 hours.

Let us assume that you had your dinner at around 8pm on Monday and you need to fast until 8pm on Tuesday. It will give you a fasting window of 24 hours. You can even start your fast after breakfast on any given day and fast until breakfast on the consecutive day. You can select the timings according to your convenience. The idea is to fast for 24 hours. During the fasting period, you cannot consume any solid food and can have all sorts of calorie-free beverages. You can have plenty of water, black coffee, black tea, herbal teas and so on. If weight loss is your primary reason to follow this diet, then you need to eat well-balanced and healthy meals during your feeding time. The only problem with this method is that the 24-hour fasting window might be a little too much for beginners. You don't necessarily need to choose this method to start with, and can slowly ease your way into this routine. You can start with either of the previous methods and, once your body gets accustomed to fasting, you can try this method. The 24-hour fasting model works well for all those who have an all-or-nothing attitude.

Alternate Day Fasting

As it is obvious from the name, in this method of intermittent fasting, you fast on alternate days. There are different variations of this method. A couple of methods suggest that you can have about 500 calories on alternate days and others suggest a strict fast. The benefits of this diet are the same as those of any other form of intermittent fasting. A strict diet might sound a little extreme, at least to a beginner. According to your level of comfort, you can modify this diet; however, be prepared to battle hunger pangs for a couple of times a week with this method.

Skipping Meals Spontaneously

There is no structured plan for this. You can reap all the

benefits offered by an intermittent fast without having to make any elaborate meal plans. This is quite an easy variation to follow. You will simply need to skip meals spontaneously from time to time. Skip meals whenever you aren't hungry, or you are preoccupied with some work. It certainly is a myth that people need to eat every couple of hours. Your body won't start losing muscle or even shift into starvation mode if you go without food for a couple of hours. Our bodies have been designed in such a manner that we can go without food for prolonged periods of time. Missing one or two meals from time to time will not do your body any harm. In fact, it will give your body a break and provide you with an opportunity to cleanse it so, if you aren't hungry, you can skip one meal. All the methods of intermittent fasting are equally effective. You can select a method that best suits your needs and your lifestyle. If you are a morning person, then you can opt for the lean gains method. If you are not too comfortable with the idea of fasting all day long, you can opt for the 5:2 dieting protocol. If you are certain that you can fast for 24 hours, then you can opt for the 24-hours fasting method. It is entirely up to you.

Chapter Three

Benefits of Intermittent Fasting

Intermittent fasting is a diet that alternates between periods of eating and fasting. In this chapter, you will learn about the different benefits of this dieting protocol.

Change in the function of cells

Whenever you restrict the intake of calories or when you fast, there are different changes that take place within the cells in your body. For instance, your body will kickstart the process of cellular repair. Apart from this, there are different changes in the levels of certain hormones in the body. The changes in hormones allow the body to reach into its fat stores. The decrease in the level of insulin allows the body to burn stored fat to generate energy. There is also a boost in the production of growth hormone. The growth hormone facilitates the burning of fat and muscle gain. When cellular repair starts in the body, the body eliminates any accumulated waste present within.

Helps lose weight

The primary reason why a lot of people opt for intermittent fasting is because it helps in weight loss. Weight loss occurs automatically when you reduce the intake of food, unless you try to compensate for it by overeating during the eating window. There is a spike in your metabolic rate when you follow the protocols of intermittent fasting. Not just that, most of the weight that you lose is from the abdominal region. If you want a flat tummy, then this is the perfect diet for you.

Reduces the risk of type-2 diabetes

A major health concern that human beings suffer from these days is type-2 diabetes. You can effectively manage and reduce the risk of type-2 diabetes with intermittent fasting. When the levels of blood sugar are high in the body, it makes the body resistant to insulin. Insulin helps regulate the blood sugar levels and when your body becomes resistant to insulin, the level of blood sugar increases. Intermittent fasting helps reduce your body's resistance towards insulin and, in turn, reduces the risk of type-2 diabetes. In fact, diabetes is a reason for several cardiovascular diseases. If you can control the risk of diabetes, you can reduce the risk of other diseases as well.

Reduces inflammation

Inflammation is the primary cause for a host of serious illnesses like arthritis. Inflammation is a natural reaction of the body towards any illnesses or diseases in the body. It is desirable to fight off illnesses or any foreign bodies in the body. It occurs when the unstable molecules in the body react with helpful ones like the protein or DNA molecules and damage them in the process. However, inflammation is harmful when the body starts to attack itself instead of the foreign bodies. This harmful reaction leads to oxidative stress and oxidative stress causes inflammation. Intermittent fasting increases the body's resistance towards oxidative stress and therefore, helps reduce inflammation.

Better heart health

One of the terrible health problems plaguing humanity these days is heart disease. Most of the health markets relate to an increase or decrease in the risk of heart diseases. Intermittent fasting helps improve different risk factors like blood pressure; cholesterol levels and controls the level of blood sugar. When the levels of these health markers are favorable, the risk of cardiovascular diseases decreases automatically. If you want a healthy heart, or if you want to improve your heart's health, then intermittent fasting is a good idea.

Chapter Four

Who Shouldn't Fast

Intermittent fasting is a safe diet; however, there are certain people who must not attempt this diet. In this section, you will learn about all those who can and cannot fast.

People Who Can Fast

Healthy adults

It is good for healthy adults to fast from time to time. It helps cleanse the system internally. There are no reasons why a healthy adult must not attempt intermittent fasting.

Children

Children up to the age of 18 don't really need to fast although, most children these days don't need to eat as frequently as they do. It doesn't mean they need to engage in extended periods of fasting. Fasting once in a while for short periods of time is safe and will not do them any harm. A healthy child doesn't need to fast. The only exceptions to this rule are children who are overweight or obese. Children need nutrition while growing up, but this doesn't mean that they keep on eating. If the child is under 18 years, then, in such a case, it is be better if you consult a doctor before the child starts any form of this diet, especially one that involves fasting for prolonged periods of time. As soon as the child starts eating healthy, there is no need for the child to fast. In fact, it is illegal for a child to fast in the US; however, in Europe, an obese child can fast, provided the child consents to it voluntarily. The child needs to be supervised by a trained professional.

Type-2 diabetes

Fasting is an effective method to reverse the effect of type-2 diabetes. There is research that backs this claim as well but, if you do have type-2 diabetes, then it is a good idea to consult your physician before you decide to follow any of the methods of intermittent fasting.

People Who Must Not Fast

The effect of fasting on an unborn fetus is not yet known, and a woman must not fast while nursing or even while pregnant. If a woman fasts while nursing, the milk produced by her body will not be as nutritious as it is supposed to be. Not just that, it also affects the quantity of milk the body produces. The human body cannot differentiate between a self-imposed fast and famine so, if you are pregnant or if you want to start a family, you must avoid intermittent fasting.

People with medical conditions

If you have any pre-existing health or medical issues related to your liver or kidney, you must not fast. If you suffer from bouts of weakness, are malnourished, anemic, frail, or exhausted, then in such a case, you must not fast. Consult a doctor before fasting if you happen to have any medical condition. If you are dependent on any medication, have a weak immune system, high blood pressure, or a weak circulation; please consult your doctor. You can fast with a lot of conditions; however, there are some conditions that absolutely forbid the individual from fasting. If a person is on any medication, then the requirements of nutrition will vary so consult your physician first.

Eating disorders

If you have any eating disorders like anorexia or bulimia, or are recovering from any eating disorders, then you must not fast. Fasting will worsen your recovery and will harm you.

Post-surgery

If you underwent any major surgery recently, or are recovering from any major illness, then in such a case, you must not fast. Fasting before a major surgery is forbidden too.

Regardless of your health, it is a good idea to consult a doctor or physician before you decide to follow the protocols of intermittent fasting.

Intermittent Fasting And Hormones

Like what was mentioned earlier, intermittent fasting can cause a severe hormonal imbalance if you don't do it correctly. Women are naturally more sensitive to the signals of starvation so, whenever your body feels that you are undereating, it misinterprets this as starvation and increases the production of leptin and ghrelin. When this happens, you will feel extremely hungry. Technically, your body doesn't need more food, but the hormones tell you otherwise.

Whenever a woman's body senses that it is headed towards a famine (regardless of whether it is intentional or not), it increases the production of hunger hormones. The two hormones that regulate hunger and give the body the signal to eat are ghrelin and leptin so, when there is an increase in the production of these hormones, you will want to eat. Also, if there isn't sufficient food to survive, then your body will shut down its reproductive system. The body will not want to procreate when it feels that it doesn't have sufficient nourishment to sustain itself. It is the body's natural defense mechanism to prevent a potential pregnancy. Your body will try to protect itself from pregnancy, even if you want to conceive. Your body cannot tell the difference between a fast that is self-imposed and a famine. It doesn't know the difference between starvation and intermittent fasting; therefore, the default protective mechanism kicks in.

There are a couple of side effects of intermittent fasting that cause hormonal imbalances. The hormonal imbalances can lead to irregular menstruation, amenorrhea in extreme cases, metabolic stress, the shrinking of ovaries, anxiety, depression, lack of sleep, and fertility issues as well.

All the hormones in the body are interconnected, and when there is a shift in the equilibrium of one hormone, it affects all the others too. Think of it as a domino effect. Hormones are the messengers that control all the bodily functions from the production of energy to digestion, metabolism and even the regulation of blood pressure. You don't want to disrupt the natural rhythm of these functions, do you? Because of all these drawbacks, you might wonder if you can still practice intermittent fasting. Well, don't let these side effects scare you. You can practice intermittent fasting safely if you opt for a relaxed approach. When you don't extend your fast for too long, you can attain your health and weight loss goals quickly. You can do all this without hurting any of your hormones.

Most women try to ignore these hunger pangs, and it causes the signals to grow louder, or worse when they try to ignore these cues and fail and then binge eat, They then try to balance it out by undereating, and the cycle continues. This vicious cycle can throw your hormonal balance out of whack.

In an animal study that was conducted in 2013 on female rats (http://journals.plos.org/plosone/article?id=10.1371/journal.pone.0052416), it showed that fasting for excess periods led to a disruption in their menstrual cycle and their ovaries shrunk as well. The male rats experienced insomnia and a reduction in the production of testosterone; however, there are only a few human studies about the effect of intermittent fasting on men and women. Most of the data is based on animal studies. One thing that the studies agree on is that fasting for extremely long periods can, at times, lead to a hormonal imbalance in women. Well, it doesn't mean that intermittent fasting is terrible because there is a solution to all of these problems.

In the grand scheme of things in your life, experimenting

with IF is a tiny bit, isn't it? For a woman, this small experiment can have a huge impact. Hormones are essential to regulate different functions in the body like ovulation. Ovulation is sensitive to the levels of energy present in the body. Think of the HPG axis (hypothalamic-pituitary-gonadal) as the air traffic controller in the human body. The hypothalamus secretes gonadotropin that releases the GnRH hormone. It, in turn, signals the pituitary gland to release a luteinizing hormone or LH and FSH (follicular stimulating hormone). These LH and FSH hormones act as the gonads, or in simpler terms, they are known as testes or ovaries. In women, it triggers the secretion of estrogen and progesterone that are necessary to start ovulation and sustain a pregnancy. On the other hand, it triggers the flow of testosterone and sperm in men. It is essential to time any GnRH pulses in the body, because, if it isn't timed correctly, then it can throw the cycle out of whack in women. Not just that, GnRH pulses are also sensitive to different environmental factors and can be thrown off course by fasting.

Chapter Five

Common Intermittent Fasting Mistakes to Avoid

Some people tend to run into difficulty with the protocols of intermittent fasting because they adopt a wrong approach to the diet. In this section, you will learn about the common intermittent fasting mistakes that people make, and the ways in which you can avoid them.

An excuse to eat junk food

It is quite unfortunate that people seem to think of intermittent fasting as a magic pill that will magically solve all their health troubles. Yes, intermittent fasting is quite an effective tool that will help improve your health and meet your weight loss goal; however, if you decide to binge on sugar and processed foods, then this diet will not do you any good. When you decide to follow the protocols of intermittent fasting, you need to nourish your body with whole foods. When your body is in the state of fast, then it starts to break down fats and damaged cells to provide energy. This process helps clean and heal the body. It also means that your body will be quite sensitive to all that you eat. It means that it is good if you eat food that's rich in nutrients and not indulge in any junk food cravings. If you don't nourish your body with the nutrients it needs, then you will feel hungry - all the time! If you want to keep hunger pangs at bay, then you need to eat healthy and wholesome meals when you break the fast.

Restrict calorie intake

A main reason why people struggle with intermittent fasting is because they try to restrain their calorie consumption when they break their fast. You need to listen to your body and eat until you feel full. Your body is an efficient machine and it knows what it needs. You need to learn to listen to your body if you want it to function properly. You needn't restrict your calorie intake. Ensure that you fill yourself up with foods that are rich in fats and fiber. If you don't consume sufficient calories, you run the risk of starvation.

Train harder and eat less

If you have never tried a diet before and don't exercise regularly, then don't try to do everything at once when you start with intermittent fasting. You must never bite off more than you can chew, pun intended! You need to ease yourself and your body into fasting and you need to train gradually. Don't train your body too hard and eat less. When you do this, you can cause severe damage to your health. Your body needs a little physical stress to function well and that's why you need to exercise, but too much exercise will unnecessarily strain your muscles and damage your health.

Obsess over timings

One of the benefits of intermittent fasting is that it will help you understand your body. When you fast, you will notice a difference between real hunger and hunger caused due to stress, boredom or other factors. You need to eat when you are hungry. Don't obsess too much over the timings. It is okay to break your fast a couple of hours early if you feel like you really need to eat. Learn to listen to your body; it does know what it needs. If you cannot fast for 16 hours and had to break your fast after 12 hours, it is okay to break your fast, but don't make it a habit to slack off.

Not drinking sufficient water

A common mistake that a lot of rookies make is that they don't drink sufficient water. Your body needs plenty of water. Water not only helps to keep hunger at bay, but it also helps the body remove toxins from within. You need to drink at least 8 (eight ounces) glasses of water daily.

Follow the tips given in this chapter to avoid the common intermittent fasting mistakes and improve your rate of success.

Chapter Six

Truth About Breakfast

If you want to speed up the process of weight loss and help your body burn fat effectively, then read on! How often have you heard someone say, "Breakfast is the most important meal of the day" or "Eat breakfast like a king!" Well, breakfast is not all that good for you. In fact, if you want to lose weight and burn more fats, then you must skip breakfast. The basic hunter-gatherer instincts of our ancestors are still ingrained within our genetic make-up. The world that we live in is quite different from the one that our ancestors were used to. There is no dearth of food in the modern times; however, the human body did not have sufficient time to adapt itself to this change. The constant struggle that goes on in between our basic physiology and the modern society is not a new one. It isn't a good idea to ignore the human physiology. Instead, you need to understand it better to improve the overall metabolism of your body.

It is a popular belief that breakfast is the most important meal in a day. Most of the weight loss regimes claim that a hearty breakfast is the trick to weight loss. Did you ever wonder where this so-called "popular notion" came from? Another common myth is that there is a direct link between skipping breakfast and obesity. Take a moment to think about it. Doesn't the idea of weight gain seem absurd when you restrict your calorie intake? There is no scientific research that backs this claim so it is nothing more than a myth and you will not gain any weight if you skip breakfast. In fact, according to the research that was published in The American Journal of Clinical Nutrition (2014), there is no effect on weight loss if you eat or skip breakfast.

Anyway, it is a good idea to listen to your body when it comes to food. You must eat only when you are truly hungry and your body tells you that it needs food. If you don't feel hungry in the morning, then you can skip breakfast. It is perfectly normal to skip breakfast. The "breakfast is the most important meal of the day" notion is a myth. Did you ever wonder why you don't immediately feel hungry in the morning? The circadian system is the answer. The circadian rhythm keeps us in sync with the 24-hours in the day and our response to light and darkness. The circadian system also governs the hormones, body temperature and the process of digestion. It regulates your hunger and appetite. The same is responsible for the lack of hunger in the morning and the hunger pangs you experience in the evening. Even if you fast during the night, you will not feel hungry in the morning. Your body doesn't burn fat when there is a constant supply of glycogen. If you consume five meals including the snacks you eat, your body will not burn any fat. If your body can easily access glucose, it will not use an alternate source of energy. If you want your body to burn fat, then you need to restrict your food intake.

Your body converts the food you eat into glucose and any excess glucose is stored within the cells in the form of fat. When you fast, you restrict the amount of glucose your body has, and it reaches into its internal stores of fat to provide energy. You can optimize this process if you postpone the first meal of the day, and intermittent fasting helps you effectively do this. It is a common misconception that your body needs a constant supply of glucose and that you need to eat every couple of hours. It is probably true if you have low blood sugar levels or if you are diabetic. If you are a healthy individual, then you don't need to eat every three or four hours. If you constantly feed your body, the tolerance towards insulin increases and it causes a host of unnecessary health troubles.

In fact, the most popular form of intermittent fasting is the one that recommends you skip breakfast. While you sleep, your body releases certain hormones that break down stored fat to provide energy; therefore, as soon as you wake up in the morning, you feel quite energetic. This burst of energy is the result of all the fat your body burns while you sleep. Also, this boost of energy will keep you going for a couple of hours so you don't have to worry about skipping breakfast and it is not as important as people seem to think.

Chapter Seven

Popular Intermittent Fasting Myths

Intermittent fasting is a popular diet. Like with any popular concepts, there are a couple of myths about intermittent fasting. In this section, you will learn about the popular misconceptions and the facts about intermittent fasting.

Myth #1: you gain weight if you skip breakfast

By now, you probably realize that breakfast isn't as important as people seem to think. It is a myth that breakfast is the most important meal of the day. It is a misconception that you will experience excessive hunger if you skip breakfast and that it leads to weight gain. You will not put on any weight if you skip breakfast. In fact, you can fast for 24 hours and not gain any weight. Your body is designed to survive prolonged fasts, and it will not do you any harm if you skip breakfast.

Myth #2: frequent meals improve your metabolism

Again, it is a myth that you need to eat frequently to improve your metabolism. It is not true that you can improve your body's metabolism to burn calories if you consume small and frequent meals. Your body needs a little energy to digest and assimilate the food that you consume. It is known as the thermic effect and it accounts for about 20-30% of the total calories you consume. On an average, only about 10% of your total of the calories consumed goes towards the thermic effect of food. You need to consider your total caloric intake and not the frequency of the meals. You don't have to eat constantly. For instance, you can have three meals worth 1,000 calories each or six meals of 500 calories each, but the thermic effect accounts for about 300 calories in either of the cases so you can fast for a prolonged period and not worry about any effect on your body's metabolism. You need to make sure that the meals you consume are rich in dietary fats and fiber. If the meals you consume are full of carbs, not only will you feel hungry quickly, but it also leads to weight gain. If you want to reduce your hunger, then you need a well-balanced diet. You don't have to worry about hunger pangs if you follow the protocols of intermittent fasting.

Myth #3: small meals lead to weight loss

Small and frequent meals don't give your metabolism a boost. Small meals will not do you any good and they will not help in weight loss. Eating frequently has the opposite of the effect you desire. You can fast for an entire day and you don't have to worry about your metabolism. Frequent snacking will not change your energy levels. If you worry that fasting leads to weight gain, then you can lay all those fears to rest. Your body will not burn fats to lose energy if you provide it with a constant supply of glucose.

Myth #4: the brain needs glucose, constantly

The brain needs some glucose to function, but it doesn't mean that you need to constantly eat carbs to enable your brain to function. The brain certainly will not desist functioning if you don't eat anything for a while, or if you fast for extended periods. It is a misconception that the brain needs glucose to function. Even if you restrict the conception of carbs, your body will burn fats to keep going. Your body starts to produce glucose through the process of gluconeogenesis. There is a reserve of glucose within the body and the liver starts to reach into this reserve to supply glucose to your brain. Even if you don't eat anything for 24-hours, your brain will function, and you don't have anything to worry about. The dietary fats present in the food are broken down into ketones to provide the necessary energy. Ketones help the brain function too. Think about all this from an evolutionary perspective. The human race will be extinct by now if carbs were the key for survival; however, if you suffer from hypoglycemia, then you do need to snack every couple of hours to maintain a stable level of blood sugar.

Myth #5: eat often for good health

A constantly fed state is not natural for the human body. During the process of evolution, humans went through periods of starvation. If it was necessary to eat constantly to survive, we might not be alive today. In fact, fasting induces the process of cellular repair or autophagy. Frequent snacking leads to the build-up of fats in the cells and does more harm than good. Any belief that intermittent fasting is bad for health is nothing more than a misconception. All the benefits that intermittent fasting provides are backed by science.

Myth #6: body shifts to starvation mode

Another popular misconception is that intermittent fasting switches on the starvation mode in the body. The starvation mode is when your body shuts down its metabolism to preserve calories and energy to function. It doesn't happen when you fast for short periods like you will do during intermittent fasting. When you follow the protocols of intermittent fasting, your body will produce noradrenaline and it enables your body to burn fats and gives your metabolism a boost as well. Fasting for up to 48-hours gives your metabolism a nice boost. If you fast for longer than 48 hours in a stretch, then your body will shift into starvation mode.

Myth #7: fasting leads to muscle loss

Intermittent fasting does not lead to muscle loss. Fasting leads to fat loss and that's about it. In fact, intermittent fasting allows you to develop lean muscle. When you combine this dieting protocol with the right form of exercise, then you can build muscle. Continuous restriction of calories for days together leads to muscle loss, but you don't have to worry about all this if you follow the protocols of intermittent fasting properly.

Myth #8: leads to overeating

Whenever you break your fast, you might feel the urge to overeat, but this urge passes, and you will experience it until your body gets used to the diet. Once your body is accustomed to the protocols of intermittent fasting, the urge to overeat doesn't last. Regardless of how hungry you feel, your calorie intake on intermittent fasting will be less than it usually is.

Chapter Eight

About the Ketogenic Diet

It is quite unlikely that our hunter-gatherer ancestors had access to carbs. In fact, the human race evolved without the consumption of any carbs. Our ancestors consumed all those foods that were readily available within nature; anything that they can hunt, gather or fish. These foods were devoid of all carbs unlike the foods that we eat these days. Our ancestors didn't eat pasta, rice, bread or potatoes. These foods crept their way into our diets only after the advent of agriculture. In a couple of hundred years, our diets went through a drastic change and our genes didn't have sufficient time to adapt to these changes. Evolution took millions of years and then a paltry 200 years ago, the industrial revolution came around. At this point, our diets underwent a drastic makeover. Factories were cropping up everywhere and, with this, came processed foods that are rich in carbs and all sorts of processed sugars. Our bodies didn't get a chance to adapt themselves to these new foods.

Sometime during the 80's the fear of fat gripped the western civilization. Fats were demonized, and all sorts of "low-fat" products started to crop up. When you start to reduce your intake of fats, your body automatically starts to rely on carbs to satiate your hunger. This is the reason for problems like obesity and diabetes to become an epidemic. Fat phobia did more harm than good, but this perception is slowly changing with each passing day.

All the carbs that you ingest are broken down into simple sugars. Your body absorbs these simple sugars into the bloodstream and it causes a spike in the levels of glucose. The body starts to produce insulin to counteract the rise in the glucose levels. The pancreas secretes insulin and it is a hormone that enables the body to store fats. When there is a spike in the levels of insulin in the body, it prevents the body from burning fats and, as a result, it leads to the accumulation of fats. After a while, the body assumes that there is a shortage of essential nutrients. When this happens, it leads to hunger and cravings for all sorts of carb and sugar-rich foods. To put it simply, it means that you will want to eat again, and this vicious cycle never ends so, when you restrict your carb consumption, your blood sugar levels will stabilize and the need for insulin reduces as well. Instead, it helps the body reach into its internal stores of fat and starts to burn fats to provide energy.

If your body has to choose between glucose and any other source of energy, the body will obviously favor glucose. Your liver stores all the glucose that you consume, but it can only store a finite amount of glucose and your body converts the rest into fat. Unlike glucose, the storage space available for fats doesn't have any restrictions. It leads to the accumulation of fatty cells.

When you restrict your carb consumption, the production of glucose reduces as well. Your body will automatically shift to the next available source of energy - fat! A low-carb and high-fat diet like the keto diet makes it easy for the body to reach into its fat reserves to provide energy. Even when you eat to your heart's content on a keto diet, your calorie intake is bound to reduce. You will learn more about this wonderful diet in the coming chapters.

Chapter Nine

Variations of the Keto Diet

There are three types or variations of the regular keto diet and they have been discussed in this chapter. These are the standard keto diet (SKD), cyclical keto diet (CKD), and the targeted keto diet (TKD). The type of keto diet that you want to follow will depend on your goals so it is a method of trial and error. Try these diets and you will be able to pick one that works well for you.

Standard Keto Diet

It is perhaps the simplest variation of the keto diet. It is usually known as SKD and, unlike the other two variations, in SKD there is no need for carb re-feeding. It is a very simple diet with a static intake of nutrition (high-fat, moderate protein, and low carb).

Cyclical Keto Diet

The CKD variation of the keto diet advocates that you need to consume some carbs every now and then to restore the level of glycogen in the muscles for a short while after the carb stores are fully depleted. The timeframe for a carb re-feed will depend on the preference of the individual, the intensity of their training, and fitness goals.

Targeted Keto Diet

The final variation of the keto diet advises intermittent periods of carb intake that are specifically placed around the workout schedule. The goal of this diet plan is to provide sufficient glucose that helps improve your athletic performance and doesn't obstruct ketosis.

Well, these are the three variations of the keto diet that you can choose from. The dieting protocol that you opt for depends on various factors. Generally, it is a good idea to start the keto diet with the SKD method. You can follow this dieting protocol for a couple of weeks, and check your performance along with your energy levels. It will give you an idea about the dieting protocol that you can select to attain your fitness and weight loss goals. You might wonder which of these variations will work well for fat loss and which one will be beneficial to develop muscle. Some people are of the opinion that CKD and TKD are ideal for building muscle. If your goal is to lose fat, then you can opt for the SKD variation of the keto diet.

However, in the long run, any temporary fluctuations in the levels of insulin don't matter as much as your total calorie intake. Here is a brief synopsis of things that you need to consider when you need to select a method of the keto diet:

SKD: It is suitable for you if you lead a sedentary lifestyle and notice that your workout performance isn't marred when you restrict your intake of carbs. It is an ideal diet for you if you don't engage in high intensity training and/or have a high resistance to insulin.

CKD: It is slightly advanced when you compare it to the other variations of the keto diet. If you opt for this dieting protocol, then make sure that you prepare yourself for a couple of runs of trial and error to determine the optimal time necessary between carb refeeds and the type of carbs that you can have on the refeed days. If you notice that your performance during high intensity training is slightly lacking when you follow the SKD and the TKD variations, then the CKD variation is the perfect diet for you.

TKD: If you prefer to train intensively a couple of times every week and notice that a reduction in your carb intake hinders your performance, then you need to add some carbs into your diet. In fact, your body needs some carbs before and immediately after your training sessions. If this seems to be the case with you, then you can opt for this protocol of the keto diet.

Your Variation Of The Keto Diet

In this section, you will learn the necessary steps to calculate your personal energy needs and the necessary macronutrient intake. It will help you to arrive at your necessary SKD intake of nutrients. If you want to opt for either CKD or TKD, then you need to make a couple of extra adjustments. You will learn about all of this in this section. The general rule of thumb for fat loss is that you need to aim for a 500 calorie deficit per day. If your aim is to gain muscle, then you need to maintain a 500 calorie surplus per day. It is a basic generalization and it will differ according to the physiological properties of your body. If you want to follow the CKD protocol, then your calorie intake will not stay constant and you need to vary it slightly.

For instance, if you want to calculate the baseline SKD macro intake for someone who weighs 150lbs while following a 2,000 calorie cutting diet, then the first step is to determine the caloric needs with the help of a calorie calculator (like the M&S BMR calorie calculator).

The next step is to set your intake of protein at 1gram per 1lb of body mass. In the given example, the daily protein intake of a person who weighs 150lbs is 150grams.

Your daily carb intake needs to be between 0.1 to 0.2gram/lbs of body mass so, in the given instance, it will be around 30grams of carbs per day. The carb intake can go below 30grams, but it must never exceed 30grams per day.

Carbohydrates and proteins contain 4 calories per one gram so the combined amount of carb and protein intake is 180gm X 4 = 720 calories. It means that in a 2,000 calorie diet, the individual will need to consume around 720 calories from protein and carbs together, and the rest from dietary fats.

The total calories to be derived from fat are 1,280 and every gram of fat has 9 calories so the amount of fat for a person who weighs 150lbs is 142grams per day (1280/9); therefore, the overall breakdown of nutrients will be 150gm from protein, 142gm from fat and 30g from carbs.

If you choose to have three meals per day, then here is a sample of a 3-meal breakdown of nutrients:

- *Meal 1:* 50g of protein, 10g of carbs and 50g of fat.

- *Meal 2:* 50g of protein, 10g of carbs and 46g of fat.

- *Meal 3:* 50g of protein, 10g of carbs and 46g of fat.

If you decide to have 5 meals per day instead of three, then, in such a case, here is an ideal breakdown of total nutrients per meal.

- *Meal 1:* 3og of protein, 10g of carbs and 30g of fat.

- *Meal 2:* 30g of protein, 5g of carbs and 30g of fat.

- *Meal 3:* 30g of protein, 5g of carbs and 30g of fat.

- *Meal 4:* 30g of protein, 5g of carbs and 27g of fat.

- *Meal 5:* 30g of protein, 5g of carbs and 25 gm of fat.

There are a couple of foods that are keto friendly and then there are those that you need to avoid at all costs. According to the type of the keto diet that you want to follow, the foods you consume will vary too. If you decide to follow an SKD protocol, the intake of carbs will be quite low, and the intake of fat will be high. Here are a couple of foods that you can consider. Have lots of animal protein (red meat to be specific), whole eggs (white only), full-fat dairy products (cream, milk, cheese, and so on), oils (canola, peanut, flax, macadamia, olive, and coconut), nuts and naturally fibrous vegetables. During the carb re-feeding portions of the diet, you can incorporate starchy and sugary sources like fruit.

Alterations Necessary For CKD

If you want to follow the CKD protocol, then you need to learn to incorporate carbs into your keto diet in a cyclical fashion. If this is your first attempt at CKD, then it is advisable that you start with a single carb re-feed every week and adjust the time between the re-feeds, as you deem necessary. The method of trial and error is the only way in which you can successfully implement this dieting protocol. It takes a lot of personal experimentation to find a carb re-feed pattern that works well for you. You need to keep a track of the carbs you consume, the type of carbs and your body's reaction to those carbs. An important point that you need to keep in mind when you increase the intake of carbs is to reduce your intake of fats. Don't stuff yourself up with fats as well as carbs. If you do this, then it will obviously lead to weight gain and not weight loss. You need to vary the intake of carbs and fats while the intake of protein stays the same.

Let us take the example of an individual weighing 150lbs. Here are some baseline recommendations that you need to take into consideration if you want to start CKD with provision for a carb re-feed once every week.

Let your protein intake be set at 1gm/lb of the body mass so, if you weigh 150lb, then your daily protein consumption needs to be 150gm.

For low insulin sensitivity, the carb intake needs to be set between 1 to 1.5gm/lb of body mass.

For moderate insulin sensitivity, the carb intake can be between 2 to 2.5gm/lb of the body mass.

For high insulin sensitivity, the carb intake must be between 3-3.5 gm/lb of the body mass.

Now, like mentioned in the previous macros calculation, simply calculate the calories that are left over after subtracting the calorie limits of carbs and proteins and you will obtain the daily caloric intake of fats. Now, divide this by 9 and you will have the number of grams of fat that you can have during your carb re-feed.

Example of a CKD for moderate insulin sensitivity in an individual who weighs 150lb on a 2,000 calorie cutting diet: Follow the SKD macronutrients breakdown from Monday to Saturday. On Sunday, the day of carb re-feed, have 2,500 calories instead of 2,000), consume 150gm of protein, 300gm of carbs and 78gm of fat.

An example of a CKD for high insulin sensitivity in an individual who weighs 150lb on a 3,000 calories bulking diet: From Monday to Saturday, follow the SKD macros breakdown and on Sunday, the day of your carb re-feed, have 150gm of protein, 450gm of carbs, and 67gm of fat.

Alterations Necessary For TKD

Now, let us look at how you can implement a TKD. Just like CKD, while you implement the protocols of TKD, it will take your body some time to get used to the changes. It will also take you a while to figure out the desired number of carbs required for a re-feed. Take some time and see how your body responds to different levels of carb intake. The aim of TKD is to make sure that you consume sufficient carbs so that your performance improves without any overexertion.

CKD helps restore the levels of glycogen, whereas TKD provides the energy boost necessary for high intensity workouts. Based on the assumption that you want to engage in intensive training for 5 days every week, you will need to consume carbs before and/or after their training sessions on those days. On the other two days, you can follow the protocols of SKD. The breakdown of macros on the TKD is akin to SKD; however, in the former, carbs are added to the meal consumed prior to the intensive training. Let us look at the breakdown of nutrients on a TKD based on the above-mentioned example of an individual weighing 150lbs on a 2000 calorie cutting diet and his/her insulin sensitivity is used as a parameter to test his/her peri-workout carb intake. Peri-workout refers to the meal you have before and after your workout. You can split your carbs anyway you feel like, as long as you stick to the time frame. It is ideal if you split your carb intake equally before and after you train.

The protein intake will stay the same; that is, it needs to be set at 1gram/lbs of body mass so an individual weighing 150lb must have 150gm of protein daily.

For low insulin sensitivity, you must add 0.25gm of carbs/lbs of the body mass; for medium insulin sensitivity, you must add 0.3755gm of carbs/lbs of the body mass and, for high insulin sensitivity, you must add 0.5gm of carbs/lbs of the body mass.

Now, you simply need to consider the "extra" carb intake along with your protein intake and the rest will come from fats.

Here is an example of TKD for an individual with low insulin sensitivity weighing about 150lb and following a 2000 calorie cutting diet: On training days, follow the regular SKD macros breakdown and add about 37-38gm carbs peri-workout. On all the other days, follow the normal SKD nutrient breakdown.

Here is an example of TKD for an individual with high insulin sensitivity weighing about 150lbs and following a 3000 calorie bulking diet: On the training days, follow the regular SKD macros breakdown and add 75gm of carbs per workout. On all the other days, just follow the SKD guidelines.

If you want to consume 5 meals on a training day while

you follow the protocols of TKD, then the breakdown of nutrients for an individual weighing 150lbs and following a bulking up diet is as follows:

- *Meal 1:* The pre-workout meal must contain 30g of protein, 40g of carbs and 20g of fats.

- *Meal 2:* The post-workout meal must have 30g of protein, 35g of carbs and 20gm of fats.

- *Meal 3:* It must contain 30g of protein, 10g of carbs and 60g of fat.

- *Meal 4:* It must contain 30g of protein, 10g of carbs and 60g of fat.

- *Meal 5:* It must contain of 30g of protein, 10g of carbs and 60g of fat.

Remember that the diet outlines and recommendations for carb consumption discussed in this chapter for the variations of keto (TKD and CKD) are just starting points. It isn't possible to provide a list of all the variables or the optimal value for every person, since there are too many things that come into play. If you want to try these variations or even this diet in general, you need to be open to experimentation, even more so if you want to try TKD or CKD. Once you start to experiment, you will realize what works well for your body. Listen to your body and learn to adapt according to the needs of your body. There is no specific guide to follow. You will need to experiment and see for yourself. There is plenty of scope for customization and there is no scientific approach to this.

Chapter Ten

Benefits of the Ketogenic Diet

In this chapter, you will learn about the different benefits of the ketogenic diet.

Reduces your appetite

Hunger is perhaps the most difficult side effect that you will have to cope with while on a diet. It is also the primary cause why a lot of people tend to just give up on their diets. One of the advantages of a low-carb diet is that it reduces your appetite naturally. When you reduce your intake of carbs and instead replace it with dietary fats and proteins, the number of calories you consume will reduce as well.

Helps with weight loss

One of the easiest and effective ways in which you can shed all those extra pounds is to simply eliminate all the carbs that you consume. It is easier to lose weight on a low-carb and a high-fat diet when compared to all the other diets. One of the main reasons for this is the removal of excess water that's present in the body. Once the insulin levels in the body reduce, the kidneys will kickstart the process of the removal of all the excess sodium and it leads to the shedding of water weight.

Loss of fat from the abdominal region

All the fat that's present in your body isn't the same. According to the location and the concentration of fat, the health risks associated with it tend to vary. The fat content in the body is usually distributed into two parts - the layer of fat under our skin and visceral fat (abdominal fat). The fat that gets accumulated around the organs is referred to as visceral fat. When the content of visceral fat is high, it not only obstructs the movement of insulin but also causes inflammation. It is the primary cause of metabolic dysfunction. A diet that's low in carbohydrates is extremely helpful to remove this harmful fat. Most of the fat that you will lose on the ketogenic diet is from the abdominal cavity.

Reduces the levels of triglycerides

Fat molecules that are present in the body are called triglycerides. When you observe an overnight fast, the level of triglycerides in the blood increases and this, in turn, increases the risk of various heart diseases. A high level of triglycerides puts you at the risk of different cardiovascular diseases. Whenever you consume carbohydrates and fructose it causes a spike in these fat molecules. The keto diet helps control and reduces the levels of triglycerides in the body.

Improvement in the level of good cholesterol

HDL stands for High Density Lipoprotein and it is dubbed as good cholesterol. Technically, it is incorrect to call this as cholesterol as it's a lipoprotein that is responsible for carrying cholesterol molecules. There's nothing called good or bad cholesterol per se because all the molecules of cholesterol have the same composition. HDL and LDL are two lipoproteins that are responsible for carrying cholesterol in the bloodstream. HDL transports the molecules of cholesterol away from the body. The higher the level of HDL, the lower is the risk of heart diseases. One of the most effective ways in which you can increase your good cholesterol is to consume foods that are rich in fats and low in carbohydrates.

Reduces the blood sugar levels

All the carbohydrates that you consume are broken down into simple sugars during digestion. When this happens, the simple sugars enter the bloodstream and it leads to an increase in the level of your blood sugar. A high level of blood sugar is toxic and the body starts to secrete insulin. Insulin helps to break down these simple sugars into glucose and transports it to different cells. The cells then burn glucose to generate energy.

Blood pressure reduces

Hypertension is a condition where the old pressure levels are unusually high. It is a leading cause for numerous heart diseases and other conditions like kidney failure. Hypertension affects all the major organs of the body and it can even cause damage to the eyesight. The ketogenic diet helps control the blood pressure levels and therefore it also reduces the risk of all the above-mentioned disorders.

Ldl cholesterol improves

LDL refers to Low Density Lipoprotein and it is dubbed as bad cholesterol. LDL is a lipoprotein that transports cholesterol molecules in the body. Research shows that individuals who have a higher level of LDL are more susceptible to heart diseases. It is also important to identify the type of LDL that is present. The type of LDL is determined according to the size of the molecules. The smaller the particles, the higher is the risk of an individual being prone to various heart diseases and vice versa.

Other benefits

The human brain needs a constant supply of glucose. A part of the brain needs glucose to function. It is the reason why the liver produces glucose even when you consume fats instead of carbohydrates. A major part of the brain makes use of ketones. The body produces ketones during ketosis. When you limit your carb intake, it helps induce the body into ketosis. It is the mechanism that the ketogenic diet makes use of, and it has proven to be successful in treating epilepsy to some extent, especially in children who don't respond to any medical treatments. In the recent past, all those diets that favor a low carbohydrate consumption have been gaining popularity for helping patients with various mental disorders like Alzheimer's and Parkinson's for coping with various symptoms of these diseases. Following the keto diet is quite beneficial for your overall wellbeing.

Chapter Eleven

How to Achieve Ketosis

You might think about how you reach ketosis. Now that you know that you need to restrict your carb intake to achieve ketosis, there is another thing that you need to do to achieve the desired level of ketosis. The first thing is that it will take a while for your body to reach the optimal stage of ketosis. Never give up on the diet if you don't achieve ketosis within the first try. This diet does take a while to work and it is a process of trial and error.

The first step to achieve ketosis is to stick to a diet that is deficient in carbs, so get rid of all those items that consist of a lot of carbs. A couple of items that you must immediately remove from your diet are starches like bread, sugar, pasta, rice, grains, potatoes and the like. You need to re-evaluate your protein intake. A high protein diet will prevent your body from entering ketosis. Once you get rid of all the carbs, the next step is to increase your intake of fats. You might think that the idea of eating fats to lose fat sounds dubious. Well, don't you worry. The ketogenic diet works on the principle of eating fats to lose fat. You need to understand that this diet will work only if dietary fats are your primary source of energy. Since it is the primary source of energy, you need to consume plenty of healthy fats. If you don't consume sufficient fats after you restrict your carb intake, you can hurt the functioning of your body and its metabolism.

So, how do you know when you reach ketosis? It is quite simple to determine whether your body has reached ketosis or not. You need to measure the ketones present in your body. There are a couple of methods that you can use. The least expensive and the easiest method to measure the ketones in your blood is with a finger prick machine that you can buy from your local pharmacy. To measure the ketones in your body, you need to perform the finger prick step first thing in the morning on an empty stomach. The optimal range of ketones necessary to induce ketosis is between 0.5 to 3 mmol/L. Anything that's higher than this range indicates that your body doesn't have sufficient fuel to sustain itself. If you deprive your body of the necessary foods, you can cause severe harm to yourself. You can check the level of ketones with the help of Ketostix and you can buy them at a local pharmacy. You need to pee on the stick and it will determine the level of ketosis your body is at, but you need to understand that this method is not as adequate as the previous one. The third method is with a breath taste. If you notice that your breath has a slightly fruity odor, it means that you have successfully entered into ketosis. Don't worry about the keto breath, it will go away in a few weeks and isn't permanent.

Chapter Twelve

Keto Food List

In this section, you will learn about the different food items that you can and cannot consume when you follow the protocols of the ketogenic diet.

Eat Freely

Protein

- Grass-fed meats (beef, lamb, goat, and venison)
- Fish caught in the wild
- Pastured pork, poultry, and eggs
- Offal (only if it is grass fed)

Healthy fats

- Saturated fats like lard, tallow, chicken, duck, or goose fat, ghee, butter, and coconut oil.
- Monounsaturated fats like avocado, macadamia,

and olive oil

- Polyunsaturated fats derived from animal sources, like fatty fish and other seafood rich in Omega-3

Non-starchy vegetables

- Spinach, lettuce, chives, radicchio, bok choy, and all sorts of green leafy vegetables

- Cruciferous vegetables like kale, kohlrabi, and radish.

- Asparagus, cucumbers, zucchini, spaghetti squash, bamboo shoots, and celery.

Beverages and condiments

- Water, black coffee, green tea, black tea, or any other herbal teas

- Bone broth

- Mayonnaise

- Pesto

- Mustard

- Pickles and fermented foods (like kimchi and kombucha)

- Sauerkraut (provided you are making it at home)

- All spices and herbs are allowed

- Whey proteins without any additives, sweeteners, and hormones

Eat Occasionally

Vegetables and fruit

- Cruciferous vegetables like white and red cabbage, cauliflower, broccoli, fennel, turnips, swede, and Brussel sprouts

- Eggplants, tomatoes, peppers and other nightshades

- A couple of root vegetables like spring onions, parsley root, garlic, mushrooms, pumpkin, and leeks

- Nori, okra, sugar snap peas, bean sprouts, wax beans, water chestnuts, and artichokes

- Berries like cranberries, blackberries, blueberries,

raspberries, strawberries, and so on.

Dairy products

Full fat cream, yogurt, sour cream and cottage cheese. You must steer clear of all those products that are labeled as "low-fat" or "diet." Most of these products have a high sugar and starch content.

Nuts and seeds

Macadamia nuts, pecans, almonds, walnuts, sunflower seeds, pine nuts, flaxseeds, pumpkin seeds, sesame seeds and hemp seeds. You can also have some Brazil nuts (however, they have a very high level of selenium so don't eat too many of those).

Fermented soy products

All non-GMO and soy products like tempeh, soy sauce and other Paleo-friendly soy products, edamame and unprocessed black soybeans.

Condiments

- Tomato products without any added sugars like puree or ketchup

- Healthy sweeteners like stevia, swerve, erythritol, and so on

- Thickeners like arrowroot powder and xanthan gum

- Extra dark chocolate (more than 70% cocoa content and be wary of soy lecithin)

- Cocoa powder and carob powder are allowed in moderation

- Steer clear of any sugar-free mints and chewing gums since they have carbs in them

Vegetables, fruit, nuts and seeds with average carbs

- Root vegetables (celery root, carrots, beets, parsnip, and sweet potatoes)

- Melons (watermelons, honeydew melon, and cantaloupe)

- Nuts (pistachios, cashew nuts, and chestnuts)

Note: Apricots, dragon fruit, peaches, nectarines, apples, grapefruit, kiwis, oranges, plums, cherries, pears, and figs are better to avoid completely, if not consume them in very small quantities.

Alcohol

Dry red and white wines and unsweetened spirits; however, if you want to lose weight, then it is better to avoid alcohol altogether.

Foods To Avoid

You must avoid all grains, even wholemeal grains like wheat, rye, corn, barley, millets, sorghum, rice, buckwheat, and other grains. You cannot have quinoa or white potatoes. It means that you need to avoid all products made from one or more of these grains.

Pork and fish that are farmed in factories. These products are rich in Omega-6 fatty acids and the fish are farmed so have a high content of mercury.

Stay away from all sugary and sweet treats. Processed and packaged foods are rich in sugars and carbs. It means no soft drinks, ice creams, sugary syrups, and cakes.

Processed foods that contain carrageenan (like products containing almond milk), products that contain MSG, dried fruit (that contain Sulphites), and wheat glutens.

Stay away from artificial sweeteners like Splenda, Equal, and other sweeteners containing saccharin, sucralose, and aspartame.

Refined fats, oils, and trans fats like margarine aren't allowed. You cannot use sunflower oil, cottonseed oil, canola oil, corn oil, grapeseed oil, and even soybean oil.

Stay away from all sorts of products that are labeled as low-fat, low carb, zero-carb, and diet. These contain artificial additives that aren't good for your health.

You can have milk, as long as it is full fat.

Stay away from alcoholic drinks and other sweet drinks. Added sugars won't do your body any good while on a diet.

Tropical fruit like pineapple, mangoes, papayas, and bananas aren't allowed. There are a few fruits that have a high carb count like tangerine and grapes. Avoid consuming any fruit juices, even the ones that say they are 100% natural. Juices contain additives and added sugars. This isn't good for your health. Smoothies are a better option and they have more fiber content in them.

Chapter Thirteen

Intermittent Fasting & The Ketogenic Diet

If you cannot decide between intermittent fasting and the ketogenic diet, you might want to combine these two diets. When you combine these diets, the benefits it offers is more than what each of these diets can provide on their own. Not only will you be able to lose weight easily, it also induces ketosis easily. Intermittent fasting promotes weight loss, controls appetite, improves digestion and detoxifies the body. You can amplify these benefits when you combine intermittent fasting with the keto diet. The most popular method of intermittent fasting is the one where the fasting window extends to 16 hours. In this method, your eating window is restricted to a four to eight-hour period. It is easier to fast on the keto diet than any of the other diets. When you follow the protocols of the ketogenic diet, you tend to consume a lot of fatty food. Fatty foods leave you feeling fuller for longer and therefore your appetite reduces. The high-fat diet makes it easier to fast. The keto diet balances your sugar levels and prevents the production of hunger hormones like ghrelin. When this happens, your body naturally suppresses your hunger. A reduction in your appetite, along with a reduction in your calorie intake, will help in weight loss.

When there is a reduction in your intake of food, the body starts to burn all the stored fat to provide energy once ketosis begins. Fasting makes it easier for the body to enter ketosis since there is no other source of energy available during the fasting period. You don't need to fast on the ketogenic diet, but if you do, it can speed up the results. When you start to fast, your body reaches into its stores of glycogen to provide energy. Once it runs out of glycogen, it starts to look for alternative sources of energy.

It is quite easy to combine these two diets. The first step is to select one method of intermittent fasting. Once you select a protocol of intermittent fasting, the next step is to simply eat keto-friendly foods when you break your fast. For instance, if the eating window stretches from noon until 8pm, then the food that you can consume during this period must be keto-friendly. Use the keto food list to make sure that you always have keto ingredients and supplies in your pantry. Go through the various recipes given in this book to cook tasty and healthy food.

If you notice any decrease in your appetite while your energy levels stay constant, it means that the combined diet is working for you but, before you try to combine these diets, start with one diet at least. You need to see the way your body reacts to a diet before you make a plan to follow it. Once your body gets used to one diet, you can easily incorporate the protocols of the other diet. If you feel lightheaded, weak, tired, extremely hungry or cranky on either of the diets, then combining these two will worsen the side effects you experience. You might need to experiment a little before you find the perfect combination of intermittent fasting and a keto diet. Also, when you decide to club these diets together, you need to take your workout schedule into consideration. On days you want to do any form of high intensity exercises, you might need to include a little carbs in your diet. If you have any pre-existing medical conditions, are pregnant, have any eating disorders or are recovering from surgery, then you must not attempt these diets. It is always advisable to consult your physician before you start a new diet.

Chapter Fourteen

Tips While Eating Out

Now that you know the benefits and the protocols of intermittent fasting, as well as the keto diet, the next step is to combine these diets. If you don't want to give up on your social life because of your diet, then the combination of these diets will work well for you. You don't have to worry about going out and not being able to eat. In fact, it is quite easy to follow a low-carb and a high-fat diet. There are a couple of things that you must keep in mind while eating out and you can make your diet work!

No starch

The keto diet doesn't make many allowances for carbs so stay away from all sorts of starchy items on the menu. It means that you must avoid bread, pasta, pizza, potatoes, rice, and other grains. Let the temptation of starchy foods stay away from your plate. If you decide to order an entrée for yourself, then ask for a substitute for the starchy side. Instead of mashed potatoes, you can ask for a portion of salad or vegetables. If possible, you can ask for a lettuce wrap instead of a sandwich or a burger. If there is something on your plate that is starchy and you didn't replace it, then just leave that item. You can always explain your dietary restriction to your server and request them to prepare something that you can eat without any worry.

Carbs aren't the only way in which you can fill yourself up. You can add some extra cheese or butter to your vegetables and, instead of a bowl of pasta, you can have a steak or some other fatty red meat. You can also ask for additional dressing with your salad but make sure that you ask your server what oil is used for the dressing. Ask them for some olive oil instead of the regular vegetable oil that they might be serving with their food. If you feel that there is nothing on the menu that works for you, then you can improvise a little. Perhaps you can ask for spaghetti Bolognese without the pasta. You can ask the server for a portion of the sauce in a bowl with a side of vegetables. Add a little bit of parmesan to it and it will be tasty on its own.

The condiments matter

There are a couple of sauces like Béarnaise that have a high-fat content and are quite rich. Then there are other sauces like barbeque sauce or ketchup that are full of carbs and sugars. Gravies can swing either ways. If you aren't sure of the sauce, then you can ask for the ingredients used in it and see whether it has any flour and sugar in it or not. Alternatively, you can ask for the sauce on the side and then you can decide whether you want to add it to your meal or not. Ask your server for fatty sauces instead of sauces loaded with sugars.

Choose your drink carefully

The perfect option for drinks is water (sparkling or still), tea, or coffee. If you want to have some alcoholic beverage, then opt for champagne, dry wine, or clear spirits. Be mindful of the quantity as hidden carbs can creep up on you at any time. Stay away from all pre-packed drinks, even if it says 100% natural.

Dessert

If you find that you are still hungry or that you want to eat something sweet, then you can indulge in a cup of tea or coffee with some cream. Good options are decaf coffee or herbal tea. Stay away from desserts. If you do want something sweet then have some berries with a side of unsweetened heavy cream, or add in some heavy cream to your coffee to satiate your sweet tooth. You can occasionally indulge in small amounts of dark chocolate (with a cocoa content of more than 60%).

At a buffet restaurant

There will be plenty of options to choose from if you opt for a buffet. There will certainly be a couple of low-carb dishes. You don't have to necessarily eat your money's worth. Eat for your health and enjoy what you are eating. Before you leave your table to take in the spread offered, set a couple of ground rules. You need to skip everything that is starchy. Always pick a small plate and you can always go back for more. Instead, focus on healthy food options like the salad bar, platter of vegetables, and even seafood options if any. You can always add a few healthy fats to it like olive oil, sour cream, butter, and even some cheese. The idea is to fill yourself with healthy food and not give into the urge to eat anything unhealthy.

A friend or a relative's place

You needn't worry about attending a dinner party or going for a holiday gathering. Your hosts will be considerate of your needs and food preferences. You can perhaps inform your host about your preference for low-carb foods, so that they can accommodate your needs. Before going to the party, you can fill yourself up on a fatty keto-friendly snack at home. It will take the edge off your hunger and it will be easier to resist starchy foods. You need to remember that it is just one meal. You can give yourself a cheat day and indulge in some regular food; however, be mindful of the amount of carbs you eat. Pass on the bread basket, but maybe you can have some fried chicken! Don't worry if you give into your cravings. It is all right. It is an isolated incident so treat it that way. You can get back to your diet on the following day and don't feel too guilty about it.

Going out needn't be a pain and you need not worry about it. You needn't shy away from any social commitments. All that you will need to do is to plan a little ahead and you will be fine. The alternative is to munch on a low-carb snack before heading out. This will help in sticking to the diet without any difficulty so you don't have to give up on your social life or your diet! They can go hand in hand. Just be mindful of what you are eating, and that's about it.

Chapter Fifteen

Create a Plan

Now that you know what intermittent fasting and the keto diet are all about, the next step is to create a plan for yourself. You must create a plan that will help you transform your body in 90 days. In this section, you will learn about the simple steps that you can follow to create a diet plan for yourself within no time.

Step 1: choose a method of intermittent fasting

The first step is to select a method of intermittent fasting. Intermittent fasting is a varied diet and there are different methods to consider. You need to select a method that suits your lifestyle, personality and your goals. Make sure that you select a method that fits in perfectly. If you like to wake up early in the morning, exercise a little and eat some breakfast, then you can select the 16/8 method wherein your first meal can be at 10am and the last one at about 6pm in the evening. If you don't mind skipping breakfast, then slightly modify the lean gains method to fit your needs. If you don't like the idea of a daily fast, you can select the 5:2 method; however, if you are comfortable with the idea of fasting for an entire day, you can opt for the alternate day fasting protocol. Before you select a method of fasting, take a look at your lifestyle and your schedule. Intermittent fasting is a flexible diet and it can easily fit into your life. When you decide to combine intermittent fasting with the keto diet, you need to follow the principles of the ketogenic diet whenever you break the fast. It is quite easy to follow. For instance, if your goal is to lose fat and gain some lean muscle, then you need to opt for the lean gains method.

Step 2: research

Go through the information that is given in this book to select a fasting protocol that will suit your needs. Before you select a diet, you need to set some goals for yourself. Once you select a diet, you need to do some research about all the things that you will need to make your life easier. The most effective diet to achieve your weight loss and health goals is to combine intermittent fasting with the protocols of the keto diet. It is a good idea to keep a few keto-friendly recipes handy. It will help you cook tasty and nutritious food within no time. It is easier to stick to a diet if you can eat tasty food so research a little and gather some recipes. There are hundreds of recipes available on the Internet and a simple Google search will help.

Step 3: necessary tools

There are different mobile applications that you can use

to simplify your dieting lifestyle. There are free ones, as well as paid apps that help you track and measure your progress. Intermittent fasting is something like the method of trial and error. You probably will need to try a couple of methods to find one that perfectly suits all your needs. It is always helpful to have an app or any other tool to simplify this process for yourself. If you don't want to depend on any apps, gadgets or gizmos, you can maintain a food journal to track your progress.

Step 4: the transition

Starting any diet is a slightly tricky process. If you are not used to fasting, then intermittent fasting might be a little difficult, at least during the initial phase. Well, you don't have to worry too much about all this and intermittent fasting is a fairly simple protocol to follow. You need to give your body a little while to condition itself to the idea of fasting. You can start with a simple method of intermittent fasting and slowly make your way through the different methods. For instance, you can start with the 5:2 method and then shift to lean gains and then perhaps the alternate day fasting method. Alternatively, to ease your transition into a new diet, you can slowly increase the gap between two meals and ensure that you cut out unhealthy foods from your diet. If you are used to snacking between meals, then you can slowly avoid those snacks and instead shift to proper meals. If you don't want to do all this, then you can simply start with the diet as soon as you want.

Step 5: necessary support

It is important to have your support system in place whenever you want to start a diet. The best idea is to find a partner for you to start the diet with. Your dieting buddy can be a family member, friend, colleague or even your spouse. Alternatively, you can explain about your diet and your reasons to choose a diet to your friends and family members. It helps to have a support system so that they will provide the necessary motivation to keep going, especially at times when you feel like giving up.

Step 6: tone down your workouts

Did you know that potency needs minimalism? Does that sound strange? Well, take a moment and think about it. What happens to the strength of coffee or alcohol when you dilute it with a little water? The potency of the drink reduces, obviously. The efficiency of the workouts while intermittent fasting follow suit. What will overtraining look like in this context? Overtraining implies training too hard and for too long. It is never a good idea to overexert yourself, especially when you fast. If you exert yourself too much, then you will just burn out and can even harm yourself in this process. Even at the right intensity, it is never a good idea to push yourself too hard for too long. It will not do you any good. In fact, it will even effectively retard your progress. It is a good idea to create an exercise routine for yourself. You can work on different muscle groups on different days of the week. You need to give your body some time to get used to the diet. For instance, you cannot bench 200 pounds on the first attempt. You need to condition your body to get used to the exercise.

Step 7: delayed gratification

Delayed gratification is a brilliant technique to keep your cravings in check. It works well with intermittent fasting. For instance, when you are about to break your fast, you might want to eat a lot of things. Ensure that you consume the necessary dietary fibers and fats before you think about eating that bar of chocolate or the scoop of ice cream that you want. Fill yourself up with foods that are keto-friendly. Once your tummy is full, the craving for anything unhealthy will disappear. Alternatively, you can make a list of things that you feel like eating whenever you crave for something. Once you get the thought out of your head, your mind will stop obsessing over those foods.

Step 8: fats need to be your priority

There are no dietary restrictions according to intermittent fasting, but when you combine this diet with the keto diet, you need to consume foods that are keto-friendly. Don't skimp on fats if you want to lose weight. Follow the principles of the keto diet to achieve your weight loss and health goals.

Apart from these steps, here are a couple of tips that you can follow to ease your transition into this diet:

Preparation

You must set goals for yourself as it is important that you have certain goals. These goals will provide you with the necessary motivation to keep going. Goals will help you measure your progress so take some time out and introspect. What is the reason for following this diet? What do you seek to gain out of this diet? What are the sacrifices that you need to make, and what will you get in return? Once you think about all this, the next step is to write down your goals. Make your description of these goals as detailed as possible. Your motivation to opt for a diet might be to improve your overall health or probably you want to lose weight. You need to review your goal daily. Take a couple of minutes and imagine how achieving your goals would feel. Will you feel proud or delighted? Will you be smiling or laughing? Take five minutes out of your daily schedule and visualize how you will feel once you achieve your goals. Make your visualizations as detailed as possible. It is a very simple thing to do. Once you start the diet, do not stop. Keep telling yourself "Yes, I can do it" and keep going.

Pick a date

Select a day and stick to it. Stop telling yourself that you can start your diet from tomorrow. If you don't set a date, then it is quite likely that you will postpone and will never start the diet. Don't wait for the "elusive" tomorrow to come around so set a date, mark it on your calendar, and stick to it. It helps if you can finalize things and it will give you enough time to prepare yourself mentally. Never underestimate the importance of mental preparation when you start a diet.

Calculating your macros

You must keep a track of your macros. It isn't about counting calories and you don't have to necessarily count calories; however, keeping a track of the macros you consume will ensure that your body is in ketosis and it stays there. A keto diet recommends a high intake of fats, a decent level of protein, and a rather drastic reduction in the carbs you consume. The ratio of Fats: Protein: Carbohydrates is around 60:35:5. One gram of fat, protein, and carbs has 9, 4, and 4 calories respectively. In a diet that recommends consumption of about 1,500 calories, you can consume 900 calories (100gms) from fats, 525 calories (131gms) from protein, and 75 (18.75gms) calories from carbs. Apps like My Macros+,

My Fitness Pal, Fitocracy Macros, Nutritionist, and Lose It can help you in keeping a track of your macros easily.

Don't forget to supplement electrolytes

When you restrict the consumption of carbs from your regular diet, your body will also stop retaining unnecessary water. It leads to rapid weight loss during the first week of the diet. It also increases your water intake. When your water intake increases, the urge to pee tends to increase as well. An increase in the rate of expulsion of water from the body will lead to a rapid loss of essential minerals and electrolytes from the body. Your body knows what it needs, and you need to listen to it. If you feel like having something salty, then listen to your body and increase your sodium intake.

Clean your pantry

Before you think about starting this diet, it is a good idea to clean your pantry. All the ingredients and foodstuff that are keto-friendly can stay, but you need to remove everything else that isn't keto-friendly. Discard anything that seems like it was produced in a factory. Don't keep any sugary or sweet treats lying around so anything like cookies, chocolates, ice creams, sodas, and anything else with sugar in it needs to go out. You never know when you might be hit with a sugar craving so always shop for your groceries well in advance. It is easier to stick to the diet when you have all the necessary ingredients readily available.

Following the above-mentioned steps will certainly make it easy to start the challenge and stick to it. Whenever you feel like you are running low on motivation, think of your goals and this will provide you with the strength to keep going.

Chapter Sixteen

Keto Meal Plan Prep

Following a diet needn't be an expensive affair. You can very well follow a ketogenic diet on a strict budget. You need not burn a hole in your pocket for the sake of meeting your health and weight loss goals. In this chapter, you will learn about different tips that will help you prep for the keto diet. You must plan your meals in advance to transform your body in 90 days.

Find a local farmer

If you cannot find a local farmer, then you can search for a local farmer's market. Instead of buying your meat from a supermarket, opt for these places. Well, it is quite convenient, and a little extra effort certainly does go a long way when you follow a diet. Here are a couple of reasons why it is a good idea to buy meat from the above-mentioned places instead of a supermarket. The quality is better, and you will be aware of what the animals were fed. Also, the price is lower. Buying from a farmer in bulk is cheaper than buying from a supermarket, especially if you want to buy in bulk. Buying local produce is always healthier. Not just that, it is more ethical as well. You can always ask a local farmer to show you around the farm.

This will help you in understanding how the food that ends up on your table is being tended to.

Buy seasonal produce

If you decide to purchase fruit and vegetables from a farmer or a farmer's market, then the produce is bound to be seasonal. If you purchase all this from a local supermarket, then you will never learn about seasonal produce. The only indication will be the price of produce. The price of produce at the beginning of their respective season is higher since not much of it is available. With the advent of globalization, most of the foods can be purchased at any given point of time. Nowadays, the availability of vegetables and fruit isn't restricted to their seasons. You can find tropical fruit and berries throughout the year these days. Not only are out of season fruit and vegetables expensive, they lack in quality as well. Depending on where you reside, make sure that you learn a little about the local produce. Make sure that you are buying seasonal produce whenever possible.

Buying in bulk

Whatever you can get your hands on, buy it in bulk if possible. Make sure that you have sufficient storage space for the purchases you have made. If not, get a freezer that is big enough to stock your produce. You can also get membership at one of the wholesale retailers near you like Costco. You need to be aware of the products that you can buy in bulk. You can buy products that have a long shelf life like almond flour, flaxseeds, stevia, and so on. You can buy meat and store it in freezers along with vegetables. You can buy seasonal produce and freeze it for further use later on. You can puree vegetables and fruit and store these, but make sure that you aren't buying any sorts of short-life produce that cannot be frozen. You can buy a couple of expensive ingredients in bulk and store them like extra virgin olive oil, coconut oil, almond flour, and other nut flours. Make sure that you are storing these carefully. If you have the time and energy, you can make these nut flours on your own at home. There are plenty of online recipes to choose from.

Shop online, use coupons, and offers

There are different wholesale retailers that offer memberships. Get yourself a membership with any of these places. You can get a membership at Tesco, Sainsbury's and the likes. There will be a couple of privileges that a membership will entitle you to like home deliveries and other special offers. If you don't want to spend a couple of hours every week at a supermarket, then you can have your groceries home delivered. Online shopping does come in handy. It will stop you from buying all sorts of unhealthy junk and you will buy only the things you need. Also, online shopping usually provides better offers than regular supermarkets. Make use of coupons and cash in on any special offers. You can always store the produce for use on a later date.

Try different websites

There are different online websites that you can make use of for buying your groceries. With Amazon Prime, you get one-day deliveries on selected items. If you are a frequent Amazon user, then you can certainly try this one out. There is a free trial period as well.

Make a list of best suppliers

This is a time-consuming task, but it will certainly be worth your while. Make a list of all the best suppliers near you. If you are ordering meat or animal products, you can use Eat Wild of Grass Fed Beef Directory (both in the US), you can use Paleo Wales (if you reside in the UK), for vegetables you can make use of Local Harvest (US), the Amazon stores of the concerned country, and supermarkets like Costco, and so on.

Foods that are close to expiration

Most of the sale items are offered for cheap prices because they are usually close to their expiration date.

You can buy these in bulk if you have proper storage facilities. If you aren't able to make immediate use of such produce, just freeze it for later on use. For instance, if you are getting a great deal on tomatoes, you can buy these, puree it and freeze it for future use.

Fasting

If you are interested in clubbing the keto diet with intermittent fasting, then you are likely to eat less and spend less as a result. If you aren't thinking about food, then the expense incurred on it will be less as well. The best intermittent fasting schedule that you can follow is the 16/8 protocol. You will learn more about this in the next chapter.

No wastage

Wasting food is not just a waste of your money, but it contributes towards environmental degradation as well. It leads to an increase in the carbon emissions as well. Did you know that it isn't the farmers or the supermarkets that waste most of the food? It is the customers who are responsible for this. Learn to make use of the scraps and leftovers. If you have cooked too much, then freeze it. Never buy more than what you can accommodate. Before you make another trip to the supermarket or the farmer's market, make sure that you have emptied your fridge and freezer. Don't buy more when you haven't exhausted the supplies that you have on hand. There are plenty of things that you can do with leftovers. For instance, if you are deboning a chicken, then don't throw the bones away. Instead, make use of these bones for making a bone broth or chicken stock! If you have egg whites or yolks leftover, then make use of these for making hollandaise or mayonnaise. If you have some roasted meat leftover from a previous meal, make a sandwich out of it or just add it to your breakfast omelet. There are plenty of things that you can do with leftovers. Learn to reduce the wastage.

Plan your cooking well in advance

Some people are capable of cooking anything with the ingredients available on hand, while others need to make plans to avoid wastage. Planning what you will cook in advance can be quite helpful. Take into consideration the dynamics of your work and social obligations. You perhaps tend to eat out frequently and there are leftovers so make sure that you are re-using the leftovers as well. Purchase the supplies you need depending on the frequency of your cooking. You can make your purchases from the supermarket, online website, or even from the local farmers depending on how often you plan to cook. Also, depending on what you plan on cooking, use all the short-life ingredients within a couple of days or see to it that there is sufficient storage space for the same! Have a couple of basic ingredients and two or three ready-to-use sauces at home. This does make it easier to follow a diet. There are several paid and free mobile applications that will help you in planning in advance for your meals. Depending on the OS of your phone, you can install a particular application.

Always make a shopping list

Make sure that you have sufficient storage space for everything that you are planning on buying. Fresh food can be left on the shelf for a while, but most of the foods will need to be refrigerated. You can leave the eggs outside, but meat and fish need to be refrigerated. Always make a shopping list before you go shopping. This will help you in buying only those ingredients that you actually need, instead of picking up random ingredients. Make a shopping list and stick to it. You can safely stay away from all sorts of junk if you do this. Take a couple of minutes and make a shopping list for yourself. There are mobile applications you can make use of. If you are more old school, then a pen and paper will do the trick. Take into consideration the list of keto-friendly foods that has been provided in this book.

Trying to grow your own produce

Yes, you can try to grow your own produce. Growing herbs is quite simple and quite inexpensive. If you have space for a kitchen garden, then make use of that space to grow some herbs, spices, berries, and simple vegetables. You can grow herbs in tiny pots and it doesn't take much maintenance. Once the herbs are fully grown, you can freeze them if you don't have any immediate use for them. You can grow your own oregano, thyme, mint, and coriander. These are quite easy to grow and taste good either fresh or dried and can be paired well with meats and sauces.

Making your own condiments

There are a couple of condiments that you can make at home and it is quite easy to do so. You can make your own mustard, mayonnaise, ketchup, bone broth, pesto, ghee, purees, and pretty much anything you feel like. Making your own condiments is way cheaper than purchasing them and you will have control over the quality of ingredients being used. You can make sausages and store these for later use. Render your own tallow or lard from meats. The list is endless. Try making your own bone broth. It is absolutely delicious and full of flavor. Collect the bones from the meats you use and store these until you have sufficient bones for making a broth. Cook these bones in a slow cooker or a pressure cooker, strain it, and then refrigerate this in ready to use containers. Bone broth can be added to almost all the dishes you cook to elevate the flavors in it. Add a couple of vegetables to a pan and some bone broth, and voila! You've got a delicious side that can be paired with any meat! You can make your own almond milk, coconut milk, sundried tomatoes, and even ghee at home!

Avoid splurging on expensive ingredients

Almond and coconut flour can be quite expensive, even more so if you have a limited budget. Instead, focus on simple eating and cheaper alternatives like eggs, meat, butter, cheese, all seasonal vegetables, fruit, and a couple of types of nuts. If you are purchasing stevia, then don't forget to refrigerate it. You simply need to store it in your fridge and it will last you for months to come. Instead of spending a lot on nut and seed flours, you can make your own ones at home. All that you need for this is a good quality blender and you can start making your own nut and seed flours, instead of purchasing the expensive stuff from the supermarket.

You can buy a bag of almonds and extract almond milk from it. The almond pulp can be made use of for making almond flour. Instead of buying flax meal, you can buy flaxseeds and blend or grind these into a fine powder. Extracting coconut milk is quite simple and the desiccated coconut or the remaining pulp can be dried and used, or you can roast it and use as a garnish.

Cook in batches

On weekends, you can cook in bulk and freeze it. Batch

cooking helps save time and energy. If you are busy during the weekdays, then batch cooking is a good idea. You can freeze what you are cooking and on a hectic day when you don't have time to cook, you simply need to thaw what you have already cooked. Cook a batch of roasted vegetables, stew, and some sauces that you can use later on.

Frozen foods aren't bad

If you have the option of having to choose between frozen and fresh foods, don't hesitate to buy frozen foods if it is cheaper. Frozen vegetables come in quite handy. Well, frozen berries are a delight, not only are these cheaper than fresh ones, but are quite tasty too.

Freeze seasonal ingredients

If there are plenty of berries available in your neighborhood, or any other fruit or vegetable, then you can freeze these ingredients. Store them in your freezer and make use of them whenever you feel like. Frozen foods are a wonderful addition to your pantry and will make cooking much easier.

Buying cheap cuts of meats

Expensive cuts of meats are quite nice. Well, don't

simply write off the cheap cuts. Cheap cuts like oxtail, pork shoulder or brisket are quite wonderful and they are cheaper as well. If you cook these cuts properly, they are quite delicious. Cook them in a pressure cooker or a slow cooker and, after a while, the meat will fall off the bone. Offal and marrowbones are cheap, and they are full of nutrients. Offal is nutritious, but if you aren't keen on eating liver on its own, then this can be added to other meats. Add this to the meatball mixture and you can add it to the bone broth!

Don't let the organic craze get to you

Organic produce seems to be all the rage these days. Organic produce is often overpriced and seldom reasonably priced. Not everything that is labeled as organic is actually sage. All these "organic" produce tags need to be accredited by a certified body and the said certification needs to be present on the packaging. You don't have to always buy organic produce. It is all right if you stick to the regular produce and don't worry about it.

Buy pasture or grain-fed beef if grass-fed beef is expensive

What's the difference between grain-fed and grass-fed meats? When a particular meat is said to be grass-fed, then that animal has been fed only grass all its life. Grain or pasture fed meats come from animals that have been fed grain or silage during winter. If grass-fed meat is expensive, then opt for grain-fed meat. You can buy cheaper cuts of red meat as well. The trick to cooking meats well is understanding how to cook them. Don't buy factory-farmed pork.

Don't buy factory-farmed fish

If you aren't able to get your hands on some fish caught in the wild, then it will be better to simply leave fish out of your diet. Avoid buying salmon and shrimps that have been farmed. These tend to contain high levels of mercury and aren't good for you, whereas fish caught in the wild tend to have high levels of Omega-3 fatty acids and other desirable proteins. If wild-caught fish is expensive, then avoid it. There are other protein sources for you to consider.

Be careful while purchasing eggs or chicken

Organic eggs are expensive than the regular ones. The common labels that you will notice on eggs and chicken are free-range, pasture-raised, or organic. You need to understand the difference between all these labels so that you don't end up paying more for something just because it sounds fancy. You can purchase eggs and chicken from a local farmer too. While buying chicken, you can buy the whole bird instead of a couple of cuts.

In this manner, you can get all the cuts you want, and the rest can be made use of for making chicken stock!

Shelf-life of oils

There are some oils that will last you a year and then there are some that will last you a couple of months at the most. A couple of oils like flaxseed oil will need to be refrigerated. Keep this in mind while you are buying oils so that they don't go rancid. Rancid oil can do some serious damage to your health. Read the labels carefully so that you don't pick up an oil that's close to its expiration date.

Coconut oil

Organic coconut oil might be slightly expensive. It is a good medium for high heat cooking due to its high smoke point. You can make coconut oil at home. It isn't difficult but it is a time-consuming process. Instead of coconut oil, use any other keto-friendly oil that is available to you. Ghee is a good alternative or even butter, and tallow is a good substitute too.

Don't spend unnecessarily on take-aways

Do you need your daily caffeine fix in the morning? And what do you do about this? You probably head to the closest coffee shop and get your cup of coffee. Well, not only do these coffees contain carbs and sugar, they are overpriced too. Instead, make your own brew at home. Carry it in a flask to your work. Black coffee and green tea are great options and are extremely cheap as well. You can buy different blends of tea and make your own tea at home. There are plenty of herbal teas to choose from! If you ever find yourself craving for some sugar-rich drink, you can make yourself a quick glass of lemonade. A glass of sparkling or still water, add some lemon juice to it, ice, and a few drops of stevia and you are good to go. You can spruce it up with a sprig of fresh mint. You can make licorice or iced tea at home as well. Water infused with fruit is a good too. There are plenty of options available.

Avoid convenience foods

If you do your meal prep on weekends or whenever you are free, you don't have to spend unnecessarily on convenience foods. Buying pre-packed salad is expensive than buying a head of lettuce. Don't take the easy way out. Don't buy trimmed green beans and just buy regular ones. It really doesn't take that long to get this job done. Stay away from all low-carb products. These products are not just expensive, but tend to contain all sorts of unhealthy ingredients. Always look at the list of ingredients before you buy something. If you don't understand something, then stay away from it.

Good kitchen tools

Investing in kitchen tools is a good idea. Always have a couple of essential kitchen tools like knives, cutting boards, a slow cooker, iron skillets, blender, and peelers on hand. A microwave, oven, salad spinner, and churner are helpful too. Refer to the list of necessary kitchen appliances that has been mentioned in this book.

Get an extra freezer

If you have managed to find a good meat supplier and can manage to get good quality produce every week and you can do so at a lower cost, then you can invest in a new freezer. This will help you in storing all the excess produce and it is cost-effective in the long run.

Share with others

Not everyone will have an extra freezer lying around, or sufficient storage space for bulk purchases. You can share your purchases with others. You can share it with your friends, family members, or even relatives. You will not only be able to save plenty of money, but can buy good quality produce as well.

Tips For A Keto Meal Prep

- You can make it a practice to cook your weekly meats on Sunday. You can pair this up with different low-carb vegetables throughout the week like spinach, cabbage, green beans, asparagus, broccoli, or so on. Refer to the keto-friendly food list for more ideas.

- Cook a batch of cauli-rice for your weekly consumption. Keep this ready in your fridge and it will certainly come in handy. It is quite simple to make cauli rice, and it can be had as a side or can even be turned into a nutritious meal by tossing in some cooked meats and vegetables along with it.

- Chop or cut fresh vegetables well in advance and store these. You can store these in mason jars or simple plastic containers and keep them ready for usage in your fridge. It comes in handy and you can toss a quick salad together if everything is cut and kept beforehand. Add some protein (bacon, beef, salmon, chicken, prawns, or anything you prefer) to those vegetables and some fat (vinaigrette, extra virgin olive oil, mayonnaise, or anything that's fatty).

- Keep some pre-cooked and frozen vegetables in your pantry. Purchase any seasonal produce of your liking like broccoli, cauliflower, green beans, kale, spinach, or anything else, blanch them in water for a couple of minutes or half-cook them and then freeze them in freeze-proof containers or zip-lock pouches. When there is a time crunch, you can make a simple curry or a stir-fry by making use of these pre-cooked ingredients.

- Cook your meat in a pressure cooker or even a slow cooker. You can cook large batches of meat and then store it for usage in the following week. This meat can be added to anything that you feel like. There are endless options as to what can be done with this meat. All that you need is some creativity and let your imagination run wild. Make use of the different recipes mentioned in this book to cook delicious food. If the meal prep is done beforehand, cooking becomes quite easy.

- Make use of bone broth to add flavor to your food. It can be added to soups or stews. You can cook vegetables in this as well for improving their flavor profile.

- Make some pesto at home and store it. It only takes a couple of minutes to make pesto and it can pretty much be added to anything! Not only can it be used as a sauce, it can be used as a spread or even serve some cooked fish with pesto to elevate the flavors.

- Make use of a lunch box. By avoiding restaurants and takeaways, you aren't just saving money, but unwanted ingredients as well. Make it a point to pack yourself a healthy keto-friendly lunch for your work.

- There are different food delivery services available. Depending on where you live, you can search for a local food delivery service that will provide you with keto-friendly meals. If you are in a hurry and have a busy schedule, then this is a convenient option.

- You must always stock your pantry with keto-friendly foods, for example, a couple of basic keto foods like eggs, cheeses, cream, a couple of non-starchy vegetables, and meat! You can fix yourself a quick meal if you have these ingredients and they are quite easy to use as well. The chances of giving into temptation and eating unhealthy foods will reduce drastically if you always have the supplies for fixing yourself a keto meal.

- Prepare some snacks that are keto-friendly and keep them ready in your fridge. Keto-friendly snacks can be boiled eggs, nuts (trail mix of nuts), nut butters, avocados, and even some kale chips!

- By prepping for your keto meals in advance will not only make it easy to follow a diet, but it will help in saving time and energy too. Meal prep is quite easy and you just need to spend a couple of hours every week for this.

Chapter Seventeen

Common Keto Mistakes to Avoid

It might seem quite exciting to start a diet; however, there are some common mistakes that people tend to make when they start a new diet. In this chapter, you will learn about the rookie mistakes that people commit while starting a diet. You will learn about these mistakes and simple ways in which you can avoid them as well. There are a couple of things that people usually face when they start the keto diet, and these mistakes can have serious repercussions on your health. If you want to achieve optimum results from intermittent fasting, then you must avoid these mistakes. If you want your body to enter and stay in ketosis, then it isn't just about cutting the carbs. If you feel like you did not achieve optimal results from the keto diet, then it is quite likely that you are committing the following mistakes:

Mistake#1: consumption of carbs

"Low-carb" is a term that doesn't have a proper definition. The meaning of this phrase tends to change from one person to another. For instance, according to the Western standards, anything between hundred to hundred and fifty grams a day is known as low-carb. A lot of people tend to believe that if they consume the above-mentioned amount of carbs, they can achieve ketosis if they stay away from processed foods, but if you want your body to enter into ketosis, then you need to completely cut off carbs from your diet. You can experiment a little with your keto diet to find the optimal level of carbs that you can consume while your body stays in ketosis. As a rule of thumb, if you restrict your consumption of carbs to below 50 grams per day, it will help your body to stay in ketosis. You need to restrict the sources of carbs and you can consume a few carbs in the form of vegetables and fruit. If you want to make the most of the keto diet, then make sure that your carb intake never goes beyond the 50 grams mark. If you feel like you have hit a weight loss plateau on the keto diet, then you might want to reconsider your carb intake. Reduce your carb intake and the process of weight loss will restart.

Mistake #2: consumption of protein

The main source of energy after carbs in a regular diet is protein. Protein is a macronutrient and it is essential for the function of muscles in the body. Protein tends to make you feel full, reduces your appetite and also increases your body's ability to burn fats when compared to carbs. If you want to follow the protocols of the ketogenic diet, then the consumption of carbs isn't the only thing that you need to be mindful of. If you consume a lot of proteins, then the proteins will be converted into amino acids and this will, in turn, prevent your body from burning fats. Well, your body will try to find other sources of energy before it decides to unlock the stores of fat present within. If you eat more protein than necessary, your body will not burn fats. If you want your body to enter and then stay in ketosis, then your diet needs to have low or no carbs along with a moderate amount of protein. The ideal range of protein that you can consume is anywhere between 1.5 to 2 grams of protein per kilo of your ideal body weight. For instance, if your ideal body weight is about 60 kilos, then you can consume about 90 to 120 grams of protein per day. Anything more than this and your body will not stay in ketosis. Your body can convert protein into glucose through gluconeogenesis so try to limit your consumption of protein and keep it within the desired range.

Mistake #3: shying away from fats

The one macronutrient that humans have demonized is fat. Most of us tend to assume that most of the calories we consume tend to be in the form of fats. Well, if you think so, then you are mistaken. Most of the calories that we consume tend to be in the form of carbs from sugars and grains. For instance, a slice of cheese has fewer calories than a serving of pasta. When you reduce your consumption of carbs, then you need to substitute this source of energy with something else to prevent starvation. Most people tend to assume that cutting carbs and fats from the diet is a good idea. Do not make this mistake. Understand that the keto diet is a low-carb and a high-fat diet. It is not a high-protein diet, but it is a high-fat diet. It means that you need to consume plenty of fat to keep your body going. If you decide to cut fats and carbs from your diet, then you will feel exhausted, weary, experience headaches and a host of other problems. Don't fear fats, as long as you stick to the keto food list; however, it doesn't mean that you consume unhealthy fats. If you have any doubts about the kind of foods you can and cannot eat, refer to the chapter on the keto food list. Stick to the food list and you are good to go.

Mistake #4: replacement of sodium

The keto diet works well because it helps to reduce the level of insulin in the body. Insulin is an essential enzyme that helps the body to store fats. It not only signals the cells to store fats, but it also signals the body to retain some sodium but, when you follow the protocols of the ketogenic diet, there is a decline in the level of insulin that your body generates. It means that your body starts to remove sodium along with water.

The main reason why people tend to lose a couple of pounds within a few days of this diet is that they shed their water weight. Losing the water weight is good if weight loss is your major goal, but it is quite important to make sure that your body replenishes all the sodium it loses. A drastic reduction in sodium can cause fatigue, headaches, constipation and even lightheadedness. The best way to deal with this problem is to increase your intake of sodium. A reduction in the level of sodium can, at times, cause a sodium deficiency. Your body needs sodium because it is an electrolyte. The best way to deal with it is to add a little salt to your food. Never underestimate the power of staying hydrated. The ketogenic diet has a diuretic effect on your body. Water is good for you and it offers plenty of benefits. You need to make sure that you consume at least 8 glasses of water daily. You can start your day with a glass of water. Since the keto diet has a diuretic effect on the body, it is important to replenish the electrolytes that your body loses so add a little salt to your water. If you want, you can even add some soluble electrolytes to your drinking water. If you drink plenty of water, you can effectively curb your hunger pangs.

Mistake #5: not being patient

You must understand that carbs are the favored source of energy for your body. If your body has to choose between carbs and fats to provide energy, your body will burn fats before it turns to fats so, if your diet includes carbs, carbs will be accessed before fats. When you remove carbohydrates from your diet, then your body will automatically turn towards fats to generate the energy it needs, but it will take your body a while to shift its source of energy. It will take a week or two for your body to shift from burning carbs to burning fats. If you are trying the keto diet for the first time, then you might experience a couple of symptoms like fatigue, headaches, mood swings and the like. The collective name for these symptoms is the keto flu. It takes your body a while to get used to the new diet. You don't have to worry too much about it. In fact, if you make sure that your body is thoroughly hydrated, and you are able to consume the necessary calories, you can easily overcome the keto flu. You need to remember that your body will take a while to get acclimatized to the diet. Be patient and give your diet some time to work its magic. A common mistake that a lot of beginners make is to give up their diet within a week or two. Don't do this. If you want to see a positive change in your weight and overall health, then stick to this diet for at least a month.

Side Effects To Watch Out For And How To Tackle Them

There are plenty of benefits that this diet offers, but your body will need some time to get accustomed to the new diet. The keto diet doesn't have any major side effects. By taking a little extra care, your body can be induced into ketosis without any difficulty.

The keto flu or the induction flu is one of the most common side effects of this diet. This usually occurs during the initial week of starting the diet. You might experience mild headaches, nausea, tiredness, lethargy, and might not be able to concentrate for prolonged periods of time. You don't have to worry about this because it can all be avoided by making sure that your body is thoroughly hydrated at all times. You can add a little salt to your water to nullify these side effects. Another minor issue is cramping of the legs. It can cause a little discomfort and it happens due to the loss of minerals due to frequent urination. A magnesium supplement can be considered if the problem gets too serious but usually, fluids and salt do the trick. Constipation is another low-carb diet side effect caused because of dehydration, loss of salt through urine and increased consumption of dairy products. Make sure to eat at least 2 cups of green leafy vegetables (raw) to avoid this problem and to stock up on necessary minerals. Ketones can cause bad breath so make sure that you are carrying some mouth freshener and maintain good oral hygiene. A reduction in physical performance, sugar cravings, heart palpitations or elevated heartbeat, shakiness, and diarrhea are all common side effects of this diet. Inclusion of mineral supplements like sodium, potassium, and magnesium by consulting a doctor or dietician will help in minimizing these side effects and make the transition easier for you. These side effects are only temporary and will subside within a few days. After these slight hurdles, things will just get better and this diet will leave you feeling great and energized.

Chapter Eighteen

Exercise on Keto

The primary source of fuel for the body is usually carbs. While following the protocols of a ketogenic diet, your intake of carbs will reduce drastically. This means that it can be slightly tricky to exercise while you are in ketosis, but there are certain exercises that you can do for improving your overall health and your energy levels too. Before getting started, it is important that you don't have any misconceptions about this diet and exercising.

It is a general misconception that exercising for longer while eating less will lead to weight loss. Yes, you might initially shed a couple of pounds, but this isn't sustainable for your body in the long run. The one thing that you need to be mindful of while losing weight is the kind of food you are consuming. The food you consume must be keto-friendly so that your body stays in ketosis. One of the best ways for strengthening your bones and building lean muscle is by exercising in a proper and a regular manner. There are a couple of things that you need take into consideration while exercising on this diet. Different kinds of exercises have different levels of nutritional requirements. Exercises can be broadly classified into aerobic, anaerobic, flexibility exercises, and stability exercises.

Any type of exercise that lasts for longer than three minutes is usually known as aerobic exercise. This is popularly referred to as cardio. Low intensity and steady cardio is a fat burning exercise for someone following the ketogenic diet. Interval training or weight training of high intensity often requires shorter spikes of energy and is categorized as anaerobic exercises. The energy required for this cannot be produced by just fats. Flexibility exercises, like the name suggests, helps in increasing your body's flexibility and also strengthens the muscles that support your joints. If there is any injury caused due to the shortening of certain muscles, then this can be easily fixed with the help of flexibility exercises. The warm-up and post-workout stretches, as well as yoga, are good examples of this form of exercising. Stability exercises help in controlling the movement and also improving the alignment of your muscles. This can be achieved by any exercise that will be classified as balance exercises. Core training will come under this category of exercising.

While in ketosis, the intensity of the workout makes all the difference. The body makes use of stored fat for providing energy during any form of aerobic exercise that's of a low intensity. Carbs will be the main source of energy during any form of anaerobic exercise of high intensity. Since fat is the primary source of fuel in ketosis, it will be difficult to perform high intensity exercises, at least during the initial phase of ketosis. You will need to make certain adjustments to your ketogenic diet so that it fits your carb requirements for exercises like sprinting or even lifting weights at a high intensity for more than 3 days in a week. A regular keto diet isn't necessarily of much help in this case. Your muscles will need sufficient glycogen for training and recovering. You can achieve this by consuming about 15-30 grams of fast-acting carbs like fruit within 30 minutes prior to and after exercising. The regular keto diet will suffice for any form of low intensity exercises.

If you like cardio (running, biking, and the like) then you don't have to worry. It is different when it comes to lifting weights though. Carbs help in enhancing your performance and they help with the recovery of muscle after training. This means faster gains and better performance during your training sessions. There are two options that are available and these are TKD and CKD. TKD (Targeted Keto Diet) is a variation of a regular keto diet that encourages you to consume sufficient carbs prior to your workout so that your body is temporarily displaced from ketosis and you have a sufficient supply of glycogen. Once you have burned all of this up, then your body will automatically return to the state of ketosis. CKD (Cyclical Ketogenic Diet) is an advanced technique and it isn't a good idea to use it if you are just starting with this diet. It is usually for bodybuilding and for competitors who will want to stay in ketosis while building upon their muscle. In this variation, you will stay on a regular keto diet and then do a carb-up for two days (usually over the weekend). You are simply helping your body in replenishing the glycogen stores for the training that you will need to do for the rest of the week. Your aim is to extinguish these glycogen stores before they can be replenished once again. Ensure that you exercise for at least thirty minutes every day to transform your body in 90 days.

Chapter Nineteen

Gain Muscle While Fasting

Can you still gain muscle and weight while fasting? Did you know that you could manage to gain weight and build muscle while following intermittent fasting protocols? In fact, most of the weight that you gain will be in the form of muscle. That does sound wonderful, doesn't it? Well, read on to learn more about it. Intermittent fasting is not about a mere reduction in your calorie intake, it is about the frequency of eating. In other words, if you want to build muscle while you follow the protocols of intermittent fasting, then you need to increase your daily calorie intake.

The primary reason why people tend to equate intermittent fasting with fat or weight loss is because of the natural tendency to consume fewer calories when the number of meals reduce. Intermittent fasting concentrates on the meal frequency and not the calories you consume. If you want to build muscle, then you need to increase your daily calorie intake. You need to ensure that you consume foods that are rich in dietary fats, proteins and fiber if you want to build muscle. Remember Hugh Jackman in Wolverine? He used to follow the protocols of intermittent fasting to achieve the ripped look.

As a result, more and more people are starting to become curious about intermittent fasting in general and in the different protocols in particular. The particular protocol to follow boils down to one's lifestyle and daily schedule as some have more time to follow the more time-consuming protocols, while others have less so the simpler, but harder, protocols may be just what the nutritionist and trainer ordered for them. More than the schedule, another aspect of lifestyle is religion. Muslims, for example, are required to fast daily from 5 in the morning to 7 in the evening during Ramadan.

Regardless of your circumstances, you can practice intermittent fasting and incorporate a great workout regimen that will allow you to build more muscle and eventually, reduce body fat. This is because muscle cells are metabolically active, i.e., the more of it you have, the faster your metabolism becomes.

The following are guidelines to help you successfully build muscle while fasting intermittently:

The later, the better

If, like the Muslims, you choose a specific time period for fasting daily like the Ramadan-prescribed 5a.m. to 7p.m. schedule, you'd be well off to schedule your exercise or workout sessions late in the evening or even early morning. Doing so helps you to get your nutrients in before and after working out, especially if you're talking about lifting weights. You can have your first meal by 7p.m. and an hour or two after, hit the weights, and eat a recovery meal before hitting the sack say at 10p.m; and then you can wake up before 5a.m. to have another meal to power you through the rest of the day. By the time 5a.m. rolls in, you've already replenished much needed nutrients and are fully charged for the day.

Post workout

In attempting to build muscle while fasting intermittently, the wisest way for you to apportion your daily calories is by putting the biggest chunk of your calories on your post-workout meal. The reason for this is post-workout recovery and calories consumed during the 3-hour golden post-workout window tend to be used more efficiently by the body, e.g., for building muscle instead of being stored as fat.

That being said, you'll need to figure out just how many calories you need to build muscle and consume about 20% of that prior to exercising or working out. Take in a good mixture of carbs and protein and, as soon as you end your workout, consume about 60% of your calories right after your workout and prior to hitting the sack. If it's too much for you, consider spreading it out over 2 to 3 meals within the next 2 to 4 hours before hitting the sack.

Taking in 60% of your daily caloric requirements may

seem too much to take in a relatively short span of time, and frankly, it can be intimidating. If you find that after several days you're still having a hard time doing so, then consider eating foods that are calorie-dense, i.e., contain more calories per gram such as dried fruit, red meat, bagels and raw oats, among others, in order for you to meet the requirement. Since calorie-dense foods have packed significantly more calories, you can actually eat less in terms of volume and still meet your 60% target. Just keep it to at most 15% of total daily calories. Fat is the most calorie-dense among the 3 major macronutrients and one gram of fat contains 9 calories when compared to carbs and proteins. One gram of protein contains 4 calories and one gram of carb contains 4 calories as well. High-fat foods can be a good way to reduce the volume of food you need without scrimping on calories.

Eat as soon as you wake up

Lastly, it's best that you eat something right after your natural waking-up time when fasting intermittently. If you're sticking to the 5a.m. to 7p.m. fasting period Ramadan-style, it means making sure you eat something before 5a.m. In particular, go for slow-digesting protein that can help you feel fuller for longer and help keep your body in an anabolic state, i.e., muscle building state, for longer during the day even without eating. These food items include red meat and cottage cheese, which must make up the remaining 20% of your daily caloric requirements.

While it's not a bad idea to throw in some carbs into the meal, limit the amount so that you get at least 35% of your daily protein calorie requirements from this meal, which is crucial to maintaining an anabolic state throughout the day. Do this with the goal of consuming only 20% of your total daily caloric requirements for this meal.

Don't scrimp on the calories

If you're doing relatively higher intensity or volume workout sessions, just make sure you consume enough calories to power such workouts. While you can sustain such workouts with low calories and intermittent fasting, it won't be long before it catches up on you and you burnout. It's just not possible because, over time, your glycogen stores will be depleted and your workouts and recovery will be severely compromised. As such, you'll need to learn to eat more food within a smaller time period and a less eating frequency to ensure you get enough calories to build muscle. Over time, you'll adjust to it and it'll feel natural to you.

Chapter Twenty

How to Stay Motivated

Now that you know the different types of intermittent fasting and the tips that will help you to lose weight, the next step is to start the diet. Have you ever tried a diet before? Do you feel that you tend to lose your mojo after a couple of weeks of dieting? If you want to attain your health and weight loss goals, you need to make sure that your motivation level stays high. Motivation will provide you with the necessary strength to overcome any distractions and challenges that you might face. In this section, you will learn about simple tips that will make sure that you don't lose your motivation.

Set Realistic Goals

If you want to maintain your mojo when you start your diet, then you need to set realistic goals for yourself. Before you think about cutting down a single calorie, you must set the right target. In fact, your goals define your success in the long run. If you set unattainable goals for yourself, you will set yourself up for some disappointments. For instance, if you set an unrealistic goal like "I want to lose 30 pounds in three weeks", you will effectively set yourself up for failure. You don't want that, do you? Set a goal that you can achieve. For instance, an achievable goal is "I want to lose at least one pound every week." The idea of intermittent fasting is to help create a sustainable and sensible pattern of eating that you can sustain in the long run. Set small and attainable goals that you can accomplish so, whenever you attain a modest goal, your motivation to keep going will merely increase.

Go Slow

The success of a diet depends on the lifestyle changes that you decide to make. These changes take a while, and they cannot happen overnight. If you want to lose weight and make sure that it stays at bay, then you need to lose weight slowly. You can starve yourself and shed a few pounds, but it will not do you any good. The more gradual and steadier your weight loss is, the easier it is to retain the weight loss. Intermittent fasting is a great dieting option, and it is sustainable as well. Make sure you go slowly. There is no hurry, and you don't have to jump right in.

Setbacks Are Common

Temptation can strike anyway, and there will be times when you might give in to your temptations. There is no harm in this, and once in a while, it is okay. The real trouble starts when you use a slip up as an excuse to binge. Call it the "I have already blown my diet, so I might as well eat a pint of ice cream." If you think like this, you will cause yourself a lot of unnecessary trouble. Treat a setback as an isolated incident and get back to your diet on the following day. After all, you are only human. It is okay to face a setback, but don't think of it as a failure. The attitude with which you deal with a setback can set the course for the rest of your diet.

Don't Try To Be A Perfectionist

So, what will you do if you polished off a bag of Oreos? Perfectionist thinking gets in the way of success more than any other factor. If a 200-calorie indulgence means just "an indulgence" and nothing more, it is okay. However, if you perceive that you have failed and see it as a reason to hang your boots, it will quickly change into a 1,000-calorie indulgence. Don't try to be a perfectionist when you start to diet. Like mentioned in the previous tip, setbacks are expected, and you must deal with them in a positive manner.

Buddy Up

Making a lifestyle change isn't all that easy, and at times it might feel like an uphill battle. Well, you aren't alone in this, and you must know this. You can find people who have similar goals as yours and buddy up with them. Different forums and groups help with dieting. You can join one such group. If you don't want to do so, the next option is to find yourself a dieting partner. You can depend on your dieting partner for some motivation, especially when you are running low on mojo. Your dieting partner can be your spouse, a family member, a friend, or even your colleague at work. Your buddy can keep track of your diet and exercise regime for you. When you are accountable to someone else, it improves the chances of your success.

Be Patient

One of the significant obstacles to a diet is the weight loss plateau. You might eat right and exercise correctly, but the numbers on the weighing scale don't seem to change. The scale appears to be stuck for some reason. Well, this is known as the weight-loss plateau, and it is something that every dieter comes across. If you face this, merely turn around and congratulate yourself for the success so far. It is a part of the process of weight loss. A simple trick that will help you to overcome this hurdle is to make slight changes to your diet. You can vary the macros you consume. Perhaps you can cut down on carbs and sugars altogether and increase your protein intake. Or maybe you can double up on vegetables and cut out all fats from your diet. You can even try a different exercise routine to see if it changes things for you. Regardless of what you feel at that point, you need to remember that this too shall pass. Be patient with yourself and don't give up on your diet. After all, you have made it so far and have successfully overcome all the other hurdles that stood in your way.

Treat Yourself

Dieting does take some effort, and it might not seem fun at times so don't forget to treat yourself when you achieve a goal. A goal can be a big or small one. It can be something as simple as avoiding sugary treats for an entire week. When you achieve your goal, you must treat yourself. The reward doesn't have to be an extravagant one. Perhaps you can buy yourself a bottle of nail polish that you wanted! The rewards you set for yourself must never be food-related. Don't reward yourself with a pint of ice cream for losing 5 pounds in ten days. It doesn't make any sense and renders the diet redundant. When you celebrate your success, it will make you feel better about yourself and your diet. Also, it will provide you with the necessary motivation to keep going even when you want to give up.

Maintenance Plan

A lot of people find it easier to lose weight instead of maintaining the weight loss. It is essential that healthy eating isn't a temporary change and it is, in fact, a way of life. It isn't a one-time project that you work on. You need to design a maintenance plan for yourself so that you not only lose weight, but you can also make sure that you don't put it back on. The healthy habits that you develop on a diet will stay with you forever, and you cannot give up on them. If you want, you can always seek some professional help to come up with a maintenance plan.

Things To Expect

In this section, you will learn about the different things that you can expect when you start the diet.

It is easy, once you get into the groove

It is easy to follow the diet, once you get into your fasting groove. You can start your day with a cup of unsweetened tea or coffee, and then keep yourself busy with work until noon. At noon, you can have your first meal and make sure that you eat healthily. Your body is used to a specific diet or rather no diet up until now; therefore, it will take a while for you to get used to intermittent fasting. Fasting isn't that difficult, but it does get easier with time. Make sure that you keep yourself thoroughly engaged during the fast period. If you sit idly at home, then your mind will continuously think about food. The idea is to distract yourself from doing so. Concentrate on your work, indulge in one of your hobbies or do anything that you like. Create a schedule for yourself and stick to it. When you condition your body to eat at specific times and not all day long, it is easier to fast. Well, a good routine cannot harm, can it, so get started and create a schedule for yourself and plan your meals in such a manner that you will not feel too hungry when you fast. Also, include a little exercise!

Hunger pangs

There is a lot of debate about breakfast being the most important meal of the day. The method of fasting that you opt for is entirely up to you. Hunger pangs are quite common during the initial week of fasting so don't get scared. Your body isn't used to fasting, and it will take a while to condition yourself to the diet. A hunger pang doesn't always indicate hunger. Does that confuse you? At times, you will feel hungry when you are stressed or even bored. It is essential that you realize the difference between actual hunger and a natural craving. Ignore these pangs and get on with your day. Intermittent fasting doesn't mean that you need to starve yourself, but, at the same time, you cannot indulge in mindless eating as well.

Benefits of exercise

When you exercise on an empty stomach, you will notice that you can burn more fat than you usually will. If weight loss is your primary goal, then you can try to exercise on an empty stomach but make sure that you don't take up any extreme forms of exercise. Even yoga on an empty stomach will increase your gains. When you exercise on an empty stomach, your body makes use of the stored fat to provide energy, and therefore it burns more fats.

Change of perspective

Your perspective on food will change when you follow this diet. When you pay attention to what you eat and when you eat it, you will eat a whole lot healthier than ever before. The diet will make you conscious of the things you feed your system. When you eat healthier, you will feel better, and your energy levels will increase too.

The scales might not take a nosedive

During the initial couple of days of the fast, the weighing scales might not make a nosedive. The weight you lose depends on several factors like your diet, metabolism, and age. You will lose some weight, but don't be disheartened if it isn't at the rate that you thought it would be. The weight loss is gradual, and you need to be patient. Patience and consistency are critical when it comes to intermittent fasting. Don't give up on the diet just because you didn't drop thirty pounds in thirty days. Instead, give it some time, stick to the diet, and see for yourself. You cannot lose weight overnight. If you think you can, then you are merely setting yourself up for failure.

Well, now that you know what to expect on your new diet, you will be better prepared to deal with it.

Chapter Twenty-One

Keto and Intermittent Fasting FAQs

How long does it take for ketosis to set in?

A keto diet isn't one that you can keep going on and off of. It will take your body some time for getting adjusted and for ketosis to set in. This process can take anywhere between two to seven days. It is dependent on the level of activity, your body type, and the food that you are eating. If you start exercising on an empty stomach, this will help in inducing ketosis rather quickly. Start restricting your carb consumption to less than 20g per day and be mindful of the amount of water that you are consuming.

How to track the intake of carbs?

There are various mobile applications that you can make use of for tracking your carbohydrate intake. There are paid and free applications as well. These apps will help you in keeping a track of your total carbohydrate and fiber intake; however, you won't be able to track your net carb intake. MyFitnessPal is one of the popular apps. You just need to open the app store on your smartphone and you can select an app from the various apps that are available.

Is it necessary to count calories?

Calories do matter. There are different reasons that you will need to be mindful of while counting calories. You will need to eat properly and make sure that your body isn't in a severe deficit of calories. Also, don't indulge in snacks that aren't good for you. While on a keto diet, you don't usually have to worry about the calories you are consuming due to all the fats and proteins that you will be consuming for filling yourself up. If you exercise regularly, then make sure that you have consumed sufficient calories and that your body isn't experiencing a huge calorie deficit.

What about eating too much of fat?

To state it simply, you can eat fat. Your body will need to be in a state of caloric deficit for losing weight. This means that calories are an important marker at the end of the day. If you start consuming too much of fat, then this will turn the caloric deficit into a surplus. It usually isn't easy to overeat while on a low-carb and a high-fat diet like keto, but it is still possible. Make use of apps for keeping track of your macros and check the amount of fats, proteins, and carbs you consume.

What will the weight loss be like?

The amount of weight that you will lose will depend on you. If you add exercise to your daily routine, then the weight loss will be greater. If you cut down on foods that stall weight loss, then this will speed up the process. For instance, completely cutting out things like artificial sweeteners, dairy and wheat products, and other related products will definitely help in speeding up your weight loss. During the first two weeks of the keto diet, you will end up losing all the excess water weight. Ketosis has got a diuretic effect on the body and you might end up losing a couple of pounds within the first few days of this diet. After this, your body will adapt itself to burning fats for generating energy, instead of carbs.

How can you tell if your body is in ketosis?

The most common way in which you can tell whether your body is in ketosis or not is by making use of Ketostix. These can be found in any local pharmacy, but you must keep in mind that they can be quite inaccurate. Usually, they will give you an idea whether ketosis has been induced or not. If the stick turns purple or pink, this shows that your body is producing ketones. If it is a darker color, then this can mean that you are dehydrated and that the levels of ketone in your urine are quite concentrated. Ketostix will help in measuring the levels of acetone present in your urine. Ketones, when unused, produce acetone. The Ketostix help in measuring the acetone present in your urine and these are the unused ketones present. The ketones that are made use of by your brain and body for generating energy are known as Beta-Hydroxybutryate (BHB) and these aren't measured by the Ketostix. If you want an accurate measure of the ketone levels in your body, then you can use a 'blood ketone meter,' which indicates the actual number of ketones in your bloodstream that aren't easily influenced by hydration or the lack of it. If you have a blood ketone meter, then the readings will be:

- Light ketosis will be between 0.5 – 0.8mmol/L

- Medium ketosis will be between 0.9 - 1.4mmol/L

- Deep ketosis will be between 1.5 - 3.0mmol/L (for best weight loss)

How does ketosis work?

To put it simply, ketosis is the state that the body will be induced into when you don't consume any carbohydrates. The body will start making use of fats for providing energy so fats, including the body fats, will be the primary source of fuel. It is not only healthier, but it is also a more efficient source of fuel for the brain. You might be wondering how energy is generated from all the fats present. Well, in the state of ketosis, the liver helps in breaking down the fat molecules and produces ketones. These ketones are made use of for providing the necessary energy. How does all this help in losing weight? When there is a deficit of calories, our body starts making use of the stored reserves of fat for providing the energy it needs. Our bodies have been designed in such a manner that they have reserves of fat in them, in case our food intake decreases. These fat reserves are hardly ever made use of and lead to weight gain. Reducing the calorie intake by cutting down on carbs helps in losing the extra kilos.

Do you worry about all the fat that you consume?

The fats that we consume can be categorized into three main groups and these are saturated fats, monounsaturated fats and polyunsaturated fats. It was a general misconception that the saturated ones are bad for health, but these fats help in improving your level of cholesterol so you needn't worry about these fats. The tricky part is to deal with polyunsaturated fats. There are two things that you need to be aware of while dealing with polyunsaturated fats. Things like margarine and vegetable oils consist of polyunsaturated fats and they have trans-fat in it. You must strictly stay away from this. When these polyunsaturated fats are present naturally in foods (like in fish), then they are good for your health and will improve your overall level of cholesterol as well, and then there are monounsaturated fats. These fats are considered to be healthy. Olive oil is the best example of these fats and they help in reducing your overall level of cholesterol as well.

What are macros, and how can you count them?

Macros is the term that is usually used for macronutrients. The three main macronutrients are fats, proteins, and carbs. Like what was mentioned earlier, calories don't really matter, but it will be better if you keep a track of these at the beginning. It will enable you to see how you are doing on the diet. You will truly be surprised about the amount of carbs that we end up consuming unknowingly. If you have come to a standstill in your weight loss, then tracking macros will be helpful. You will be able to pinpoint at the different things in your diet that might be causing this. You will start thinking in terms of grams when you start tracking your macros. You must not think in terms of % and think in terms of grams. For instance, a lot of people think that 75% fat, 20% protein, and 5% carbs is good, but that's not the case. Grams will help you in getting an accurate description of what you are eating. You needn't worry if you are off by a bit on your macros; it really isn't a big deal. There is a wiggle room for about 10-15 grams of fats as well as proteins in most of the cases. You needn't worry if you go a little over or a little under on some days. If you are keeping track of your calories and it isn't too much in deficit, then you are doing fine.

What can be done if you feel a little low during the initial phase of the diet?

During the initial phase of the keto diet, you might experience mild headaches and feel a little low on energy as well. Ketosis has got a diuretic effect on the body and this results in an increase in the urge to urinate more than usual. Added to this, our bodies are burning up the glycogen stores, and you have a minor problem on your hand. The electrolytes are being pushed out of your body so you will need to replace them. Keep yourself fully hydrated. Add a little salt to your food. Consume plenty of broths, and have lots of water. The transition into ketosis will be quite simple and you can make it easy on yourself by staying hydrated.

What can you do if you experience constipation?

Your bowel movements might undergo a change while starting out on keto. You might or might not experience constipation. Here are a few things that you can do for restoring normalcy to your bowel movements. Add in a magnesium supplement, drink lots of water and a tablespoon of coconut oil will also help. In case you eat nuts, then stop doing so for a while, consume fibrous vegetables, chia or flax seeds also help, and you can try some coffee or some tea.

Is alcohol permitted?

You can consume alcohol while on the ketogenic diet, but be mindful of the amount of alcohol you consume. Alcohol is a really good source of carbs to creep in to your diet. You must pay attention to the liquor that you drink. Wine, beer, and different cocktails have carbs in them so clear liquor is a safe bet but stay away from all sorts of flavored liquors since they have carbs in them as well.

What to do if you stop losing weight?

You might have reached a standstill in your weight loss. There are a lot of reasons that can contribute to this. You can do a couple of things for resuming your weight loss. Cut down a few things from your diet or you can change your eating pattern as well. Here are a few suggestions that you can make use of. You can try any of the following strategies: cut down on dairy, increase your fat intake, decrease the intake of carbs, stop consuming nuts, cut out gluten, no artificial sweeteners, watch out for additional carbs, cut down on processed foods, and switch to measuring yourself instead of weighing yourself.

What about working out?

People who exercise can be broadly categorized into those who run and those who lift weights. If you like cardio (running, biking, and the like) then you don't have to worry. It is different when it comes to lifting weights though. Carbs do help in your performance and they help with the recovery of muscle as well. This means faster gains, and better performance during your training sessions. There are two options you have and these are TKD and CKD. TKD stands for Targeted Keto Diet. In this, you will consume sufficient carbs prior to your workout so that your body is temporarily displaced from ketosis for the duration of the workout and you have a sufficient supply of glycogen. Once you have burned all of this up, then your body will return to the state of ketosis. CKD stands for Cyclical Ketogenic Diet. It is an advanced technique. Don't attempt to use it if you are just getting started with the keto diet. This is usually for bodybuilding and for competitors who want to stay in ketosis while building up on their muscle. In this, you will stay on a regular keto diet and then do a carb-up for two days (usually over the weekend). In this method, you are simply helping your body in replenishing the glycogen stores for the training that you will need to do for the rest of the week. Your aim is to extinguish these glycogen stores before they can be replenished once again.

Will fasting lead to an increase in fat storage? Will the body enter into starvation mode?

If you keep eating after every two or three hours from the time you wake up until you go to sleep at night, you are effectively suppressing the process of burning fat. Your body never gets a chance to burn anything else apart from all the food that you are constantly consuming and it makes fat loss quite difficult. Fasting helps in reducing your insulin levels and this is good for promoting lipolysis. Lipolysis is the process through which your body starts burning all the stored fat. When you are fasting, your body burns fat. When you eat, your body is busy breaking down the food you are consuming so you don't have to worry about your metabolism slowing down and your body does not enter into a starvation mode.

Isn't it necessary to eat every couple of hours to maintain stable blood sugar levels? No. Unless you have hypoglycemia, you don't have to worry about feeling light-headed if you don't eat every couple of hours. Skipping breakfast won't do you any harm. As mentioned in an earlier chapter, this is nothing more than a myth that you needn't worry about. Our bodies have been designed in such a way that we can go on for a couple of days without worrying about running out of fuel to survive.

What to eat while following this diet?

This diet doesn't prescribe any dietary restrictions per se. You need to be mindful of when you are eating and not what you are eating while following any of the intermittent dieting protocols, but this doesn't mean that you fast for 16 hours in a day and then fill yourself up with all sorts of processed junk food. Doing this will simply defeat the purpose of dieting altogether. There are no dietary restrictions and you don't have to count calories, but this doesn't mean that you eat food that will promote weight gain. Have a well-balanced meal that's full of the necessary nutrients and dietary fiber that will keep you feeling full. Make sure that you fill yourself up with all this before having some dessert. Your meal must be rich in protein, dietary fats, and fiber.

What are the side effects of this diet?

There aren't any serious side effects of this diet that you need to worry about. You might feel light-headed and might experience mild headaches, but this is a sign that your body is getting used to intermittent fasting and it isn't something that you must worry about. Always make sure that your body is thoroughly hydrated. One more thing that you need to keep in mind is to always listen to your body. If you are feeling hungry before your fasting period ends, it is perfectly okay. Don't beat yourself up about it. Break your fast and eat something. Your body knows when it needs food and it is good to listen to it. Don't think of this as a major setback; instead, treat it as an isolated incident and you can get back to your diet from the following day. Don't be too hard on yourself.

How long does it take to get used to fasting?

It will take your body a week or two to get used to intermittent fasting. Once your body gets used to this method of dieting, you can resume your exercising schedule. Make sure that your exercising schedule isn't too stressful during the first two weeks.

What are the benefits of this diet?

Fasting has many benefits to offer that go well beyond weight loss. Fasting can help in improving your overall health and improve the longevity of your life as well. In a recent study that was conducted to study the link between cell metabolism and fasting, it was found that fasting periodically can help in decreasing the risk of heart diseases, diabetes, aging, and so on. Fasting is effective because during this period, a lot of cells that are present in the body die and the stem cells start working. This starts the regeneration process and produces new cells. Other studies also show that it helps in reducing the amount of bad cholesterol or LDL present in the blood.

How to keep hunger at bay while following this diet?

If you have just started your intermittent diet, you will probably have trouble trying to curb your thoughts about hunger. You may sit around and begin to wonder about how hungry you are and you will probably crave for some form of food so let me give you a certain pattern that you can use during the first few days of your fast! Right before the first few hours of your fast, you must consume a huge meal! An extremely huge meal, and let us call it a monster meal. You will stop worrying about when you are going to eat next! You can try to sleep a decent amount of time since you cannot worry about hunger when you are dreaming! Try to keep yourself busy during the day to avoid worrying about your hunger. Last, but never the least, keep telling yourself that you do not need to think about hunger since you are a strong person!

Is it okay to consume certain beverages while fasting?

Yes, you can have certain beverages while fasting, but make sure that there aren't any added calories in these drinks which means you will need to stay away from sodas and all sugary drinks. You can have calorie-free drinks like green tea, herbal teas, black coffee, or pretty much anything that doesn't have any calories in it. Make sure that you are drinking plenty of water and that your body is thoroughly hydrated. Watch out for the extra calories in milk and sugar. It might seem like a tough call to drink your morning coffee black, but you will get used to it, especially when you start to see the benefits of your intermittent fasting regime kicking in. Adding a bit of cream here, a spot of sugar there, or even a bit of honey can have the effect of breaking the fast and sending your insulin levels back up. That means your body is not getting the full benefit of the fast. If you are doing a 24 hour fast, keep in mind that this is only for one or two days of the week so be strong about it and push on. If you are keen about losing weight, then you need to stay away from alcohol. Alcohol is rich in calories and it leads to unnecessary calorie consumption. If you feel like drinking, then stick to clear spirits or a glass of dry red or white wines, but that's about it. Don't overindulge in alcohol because this just prevents the process of weight loss.

Chapter Twenty-Two

Additional Tips for Weight Loss

Water, water, and more water

It is quintessential that you keep your body thoroughly hydrated while you follow a diet. Water helps to hydrate your body, clear your skin, flush out toxins, and even fill you up. You must have at least eight glasses (20-ounces each) of water daily. Regardless of the intermittent fasting protocol that you want to follow, you need to have plenty of water. Whenever you feel slightly hungry, have a glass of water, and it will keep your hunger at bay. Always carry a water bottle with you. Add a couple of lemon slices and mint leaves to make detox water.

Eat slowly

Whenever you eat, you need to eat slowly. Don't be in a rush to stuff yourself up with food. When you end your fast, you might feel the urge to binge on food, but you need to refrain from doing so. Thoroughly chew your food before you swallow.

Eat healthily

Intermittent fasting places stress on when you eat and not what you eat, but it certainly doesn't mean that you eat anything and everything. You do want to lead a healthy life and lose weight, don't you? If yes, then you need to be prudent about your diet. Be mindful of what you eat and don't binge on any junk food. The food you consume during your eating window must provide your body with all the nourishment that it needs.

Cook at home

Try to cook at home as much as you can. If you don't buy any prepacked meals, you can considerably reduce your food bill. It might be easy to order a salad, but it will prove to be expensive in the long run. Unlike the other fad diets, you don't need to buy any fancy ingredients while you follow intermittent fasting. Cook at home and make sure that you eat what you cook at home. If not, it will only defeat the purpose.

Ration your portions

You have to control the proportions of your meals. You can do this by simply measuring what you eat. Use weighing scales when you portion your meals. Your meals must be rich in protein and fiber, while low in fats and carbs. Eat plenty of protein and fiber, and your body will receive all the nutrients that it needs.

Plan your meals

With intermittent fasting, you can choose your eating window. When you know the eating schedule, you can efficiently plan your meals. If you plan your meals, it will reduce the chances of wanting to eat out. If you know that you will fast the entire day, make sure that you have a meal waiting for you at home.

Grocery shopping

Whenever you decide to shop for groceries, make a list of all the ingredients you will need. Don't buy any junk food. If you don't store any junk food at home, it becomes easier to eat healthily. Out of sight, out of mind, so keep your pantry stocked with healthy ingredients. Clean your cupboard of all sorts of sugary carbs. Also, don't shop when you are hungry. When you buy while you are hungry, it is quite likely that you will give into your urges to eat unhealthy foods. If you have all the ingredients you need to cook healthy meals, it is easier to cook. When you can plan and cook ahead, you can save yourself a lot of money.

Meal prep

You need to do basic meal prep on the weekends and prepare for the week that lies ahead. Meal prep can be something as simple as cooking a stew and freezing it. Cut and portion of the protein and vegetables you need. It helps to reduce your cooking time, and you can whip up a healthy meal in no time. When you cook in batches, you tend to save some money as well. Merely freeze whatever you cook and heat it up before you eat. You can even pack your meals and freeze them. For instance, you can make the paste for curries and store them. Whenever you need to eat, you simply need to heat the curry and add the other ingredients you want.

Eat fruit for dessert

If you have a sweet tooth, it might feel challenging to give up on desserts so, to satiate your sweet cravings, you can have fruit for dessert. A cup of strawberries with a tablespoon of unsweetened whipped cream is a tasty dessert. Have berries or any other fruit that you want. Fruit is good for your body and is full of nutrients, but you must be mindful of the hidden calories they consist. You cannot have two or three mangoes just because it is a fruit. Eat healthily! For instance, frozen bananas with some peanut butter, or apple wedges with peanut butter make for a tasty sweet treat. There are plenty of healthy alternatives for desserts so try them out.

Food budget

You need to set a weekly or a monthly food budget for yourself. Not just set a budget, but you must follow it as well. When you plan your meals, you can efficiently allocate a weekly budget for yourself. It will help you to keep track of the expenses you incur on your groceries and other purchases.

Eat the healthy stuff first

When you break your fast, you will want to gorge on all sorts of foods, but the idea is to eat healthily so make sure that you have all the healthy foods before you think about eating anything that's not healthy. If you want a piece of chocolate or a scoop of ice cream, make sure that you fill yourself up with all the veggies and proteins that your body needs before you think about dessert. In this manner, you will not feel like you denied yourself a treat when you feel full.

Brush your teeth after eating

It is a healthy habit to brush your teeth before you go to sleep at night. Make sure that you brush your teeth after dinner. In a way, it is a signal to your body that you are done with the meals for any given day. It helps on a psychological level.

Don't leave the house hungry

How often do you buy coffee for yourself in the morning? Coffee might help to wake you up, but over a period, the amount you spend on your morning fix-me ups can be expensive. Why don't you make coffee at home and carry it with you? It is quite simple, and it will help you to save some money on the side. Also, never leave home hungry. When you are hungry, you will feel like eating a lot of things that will not do your health or your bank balance any good. Instead, have a light snack before you leave.

Make your snacks

You don't have to buy diet snacks anymore. You can make your own 100-calorie snacks at home and carry them with you. You can whip up healthy, tasty, and low-cal treats at home. For instance, you can make popcorn and store it up in small bags or containers. It can be your go-to snack. Similarly, kale chips are quite easy to make and are rather tasty. There are various options to choose from!

Track what you eat

You can maintain a food journal or use one of the food tracking apps to keep tabs on what you eat. The key is to make a list of everything that you eat. It will help you to eat healthily and cut down on any mindless snacking.

Exercise

You don't need a gym membership to exercise. There are different ways in which you can exercise without going to the gym. Different no-cost exercise options include jogging, running, doing yoga at home, dancing, and pure strength training exercises. Power up your laptop, pull up a few exercise videos, and exercise from the comfort of your living room!

Chapter Twenty Three

Meal Plan

A link to each recipe is available in the sources section at the end of this book.

Day 1

- Breakfast – Scrambled Eggs
- Lunch – Keto Asian Cabbage Stir Fry
- Snack – Bell Pepper with Cheese
- Dinner – Keto Fried Chicken with Broccoli and Butter

Day 2

- Breakfast – Oatmeal with Roasted Almonds
- Lunch – Chicken and Zucchini Casserole

- Snack – Cheese Crackers
- Dinner – Ham and Cheese Pizza with Asparagus

Day 3

- Breakfast – Parsley Quiche
- Lunch – Ham and Cheese Pizza with Asparagus
- Snack – Bresaola Air Cured Beef
- Dinner – Lettuce Turkey Wraps

Day 4

- Breakfast – Cheddar Muffin
- Lunch – Buffalo Chicken with Paprika Mayo and Butter-Fried Cabbage
- Snack – Peanut Butter Smoothie
- Dinner – Keto Thai Fish with Curry and Coconut

Day 5

- Breakfast – Chia Pudding
- Lunch – Keto Thai Fish with Curry and Coconut
- Snack – Spicy Goat Cheese Balls
- Dinner – Keto Pizza

Day 6

- Breakfast – Strawberry Protein Smoothie
- Lunch – Keto Pizza
- Snack – Greek Yoghurt with Berries
- Dinner – Keto Chicken Fajita Bowl

Day 7

- Breakfast – Scrambled Eggs
- Lunch – Bacon-Wrapped Keto Burgers
- Snack – Smoked Salmon Avocado Rolls

- Dinner – <u>Grilled Salmon</u>

Conclusion

I want to thank you once again for purchasing this book. I hope it proved to be an informative and an enjoyable read.

The two best diets to improve your overall health, and lose weight as well as fat, are ketogenic diet and intermittent fasting. If you combine these diets, then you can speed up the process of weight and fat loss. By now, you realize how effective these diets are, don't you? Use the information in this book to create a diet that works well for you and fits your lifestyle. The first step is to select a method of intermittent fasting that fits your needs. Once you do this, the next step is to merely combine the fasting protocols with that of the keto diet. Whenever you break your fast, ensure that the foods you eat are keto-friendly. Use the keto-friendly food list and the meal prep ideas to make the diet easier for you. Always stock your pantry with keto-friendly ingredients. Once you have the necessary ingredients, it is quite easy to whip up tasty and nutritious food.

Now, all you need to do is get started with this diet. You can see a positive change in your weight and health within 90 days. Learn to be patient, and follow the protocols of these diets carefully.

Thank you, and all the best!

Sources

Content

https://www.ruled.me/guide-keto-diet/

https://thrivestrive.com/keto-benefits/

https://www.ruled.me/ketogenic-diet-food-list/

https://www.dietdoctor.com/intermittent-fasting

https://www.healthline.com/nutrition/10-health-benefits-of-intermittent-fasting

http://romanfitnesssystems.com/articles/intermittent-fasting-faq/

https://www.ruled.me/ketogenic-diet-faq/

https://www.ruled.me/complete-guide-exercise-ketogenic-diet/

https://dailyburn.com/life/health/intermittent-fasting-exercise-weight-loss/

https://ketodietapp.com/Blog/lchf/Types-of-Ketogenic-Diets-and-the-KetoDiet-Approach

Recipes

Scrambled Eggs (https://www.dietdoctor.com/recipes/scrambled-eggs)

Keto Asian Cabbage Stir Fry (https://www.eatthismuch.com/recipe/view/keto-asian-cabbage-stir-fry,904286/)

Bell Pepper with cheese (https://www.thespruceeats.com/cheese-stuffed-sweet-bell-peppers-recipe-1136360)

Keto Fried Chicken with Broccoli and Butter (https://www.dietdoctor.com/recipes/keto-fried-chicken-broccoli-butter)

Oatmeal with roasted almonds (https://barefeetinthekitchen.com/simple-homemade-almond-and-oats-granola-recipe/)

Chicken and Zucchini Casserole (https://www.tasteofhome.com/recipes/chicken-zucchini-casserole/)

Cheese Crackers (https://www.foodnetwork.com/recipes/ree-drummond/homemade-cheddar-crackers-3141125)

Ham and Cheese Pizza with Asparagus (https://www.foodandwine.com/recipes/pizza-with-asparagus-and-smoked-ham)

Parsley Quiche (https://www.sunset.com/recipe/fava-leaf-parsley-quiche)

Ham and Cheese Pizza with Asparagus (https://www.foodandwine.com/recipes/pizza-with-asparagus-and-smoked-ham)

Bresaola air cured Beef (https://honest-food.net/bresaola-recipe/)

Lettuce Turkey Wraps (https://www.foodnetwork.com/recipes/melissa-darabian/turkey-lettuce-wraps-recipe-2041422)

Cheddar Muffin (https://www.allrecipes.com/recipe/239856/cheddar-cheese-muffins/)

Buffalo Chicken with Paprika Mayo and Butter-Fried Cabbage (https://www.dietdoctor.com/recipes/buffalo-chicken-paprika-mayo-butter-fried-cabbage)

Peanut Butter Smoothie (https://www.allrecipes.com/recipe/221261/peanut-butter-banana-smoothie/)

Keto Thai fish with curry and coconut (https://www.mealgarden.com/recipe/keto-thai-fish-with-curry-and-coconut/)

Chia Pudding (https://www.eatingbirdfood.com/basic-chia-seed-pudding/)

Keto Thai fish with curry and coconut (https://www.mealgarden.com/recipe/keto-thai-fish-with-curry-and-coconut/)

Spicy Goat cheese balls (https://www.myrecipes.com/recipe/goat-cheese-poppers-honey)

Keto Pizza (https://www.dietdoctor.com/recipes/keto-pizza)

Strawberry Protein Smoothie (https://www.asweetpeachef.com/strawberry-protein-shake/)

Keto Pizza (https://www.dietdoctor.com/recipes/keto-pizza)

Greek Yoghurt with berries (https://www.skinnytaste.com/greek-yogurt-with-berries-nuts-and/)

Keto chicken fajita bowl (https://www.dietdoctor.com/cooking-keto-chicken-fajita-bowl)

Scrambled Eggs (https://www.dietdoctor.com/recipes/scrambled-eggs)

Bacon Wrapped Keto Burgers (https://lowcarbediem.com/bacon-wrapped-keto-burgers/)

Smoked Salmon Avocado Rolls (https://www.myrecipes.com/recipe/smoked-salmon-avocado-hand-rolls)

Grilled Salmon (https://www.allrecipes.com/recipe/12720/grilled-salmon-i/)

Thank You!

Before you go, we would like to thank you for purchasing a copy of our book. Out of the dozens of books you could have picked over ours, you decided to go with this one and for that we are very grateful.

We hope you enjoyed reading it as much as we enjoyed writing it! We hope you found it very informative.

We would like to ask you for a small favor. <u>Could you please take a moment to leave a review for this book on Amazon?</u>

Your feedback will help us continue to write more books and release new content in the future!

Printed in Poland
by Amazon Fulfillment
Poland Sp. z o.o., Wrocław